Curing Madness?

Curing Madness?

A Social and Cultural History of Insanity in Colonial North India, 1800–1950s

Shilpi Rajpal

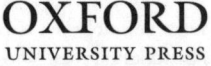
OXFORD
UNIVERSITY PRESS

OXFORD
UNIVERSITY PRESS

Oxford University Press is a department of the University of Oxford.
It furthers the University's objective of excellence in research, scholarship,
and education by publishing worldwide. Oxford is a registered trademark of
Oxford University Press in the UK and in certain other countries.

Published in India by
Oxford University Press
22 Workspace, 2nd Floor, 1/22 Asaf Ali Road, New Delhi 110002, India

First Edition published in 2021

ISBN-13 (print edition): 978-0-19-012801-2
ISBN-10 (print edition): 0-19-012801-1

ISBN-13 (eBook): 978-0-19-099332-0
ISBN-10 (eBook): 0-19-099332-4

Every effort has been made to trace the copyright holders of Images 5.2 and 5.3 on
pages 212 and 224 respectively. The publisher would be pleased to hear from the
copyright owner so that proper acknowledgement can be made in future editions.

Typeset in Adobe Jenson Pro 10.7/13.3
by Tranistics Data Technologies, Kolkata 700 091
Printed in India by Rakmo Press, New Delhi 110 020

For
Biswamoy Pati
This book is for you…

Contents

Figures and Table

Figures

Table

Acknowledgements

This book culminates a long journey which would not have been possible without the contributions of various individuals. The present work is based on my doctoral thesis, which has now taken a more definitive shape in the form of a monograph. At the very outset, I would first like to thank my mentors. I sincerely thank my supervisor Professor Amar Farooqui for his erudition, patience, and dedication. I am equally grateful to Dr Biswamoy Pati, who was a constant source of fortitude, energy, and affection and whose untimely death has left us in shock. This book would not have been conceivable without his encouragement and faith in my abilities. He had a rare quality of carving scholars out of students.

As a young student I was introduced to history by my school teacher Ms Maninder Kaur, whose encouragement helped me in transforming my teenage infatuation with history into a lifelong interest, further nurtured by teachers at Sri Venkateswara College, University of Delhi, who helped me lay my foundational understanding of history. During my master's degree, I was first oriented to the rigours of historical research. Professor Shahid Amin familiarized me with the archives, Professor Dilip Menon introduced me to novel ideas, Dr Prabhu Mohapatra to intellectual depth, Dr Anshu Malhotra to critical insight, Professor Amar Farooqui to historical acumen, and Professor Basudev Chatterjito ever striving for appropriate historical understanding. I am thankful to Professor Mahesh Rangarajan for encouraging me at several stages of this book. I am truly indebted to all the faculty members of the Department of History, University of Delhi. I sincerely acknowledge the support of my PhD examiner, Professor Deepak Kumar. His guidance has helped me from time to time. I am also grateful to Professor Waltraud Ernst who gave me an important opportunity to do archival research in the United Kingdom, from which this book has hugely benefitted.

I am indebted to people at the personal and the professional levels who helped me during the field visits to various places in north India. Mr Mohinuddin Farooqui provided me with archival material at the Patiala State Archives. Dr Kusum Chauhan at the Agra Mental Hospital facilitated the process of my gaining access to the patient case registers. I also thank the staff of the Government Medical College Library, Amritsar, for their generous help, and Ms Meena Khare who aided in providing records at the Bareilly Mental Hospital.

I thank Ms Seema Mathur and Mr Arun Mathur for their warm hospitality during my fieldwork in Lucknow. I also thank Professor S. Gajnani, Mritunjay Kumar, Professor Sukhdev Sohal, and Professor Abhay Kumar Singh for my stay in Patiala, Chandigarh, Amritsar, and Bareilly respectively. I sincerely acknowledge the help of Dr Padma Misra, Professor Sunita Pathania, Dhrub Kumar Singh, and Dr Ranjana Sheel at Varanasi.

Major parts of this books have been written accessing sources from libraries in India and Britain, and for this research work I would like to thank the staff of the Central Reference Library in Kolkata and the Ratan Tata Library, Parthasarthi Gupta Library, Central Secretariat Library, Nehru Memorial Museum & Library, National Archives of India, Delhi Archives, and National Medical Library, all in New Delhi. The staff at the Wellcome Library and the British Library in London were extremely helpful in providing me with the sources I needed.

I am grateful to Dr V. Rajesh and the Indian Institute of Science Education and Research, Mohali, for providing the much-needed funding and intellectual support in the final stages of this book. The Charles Wallace India Trust Research Grant made my visit to England possible, which further enhanced the source base of this work. Professor Sonu Shamdasani's warm welcome to the informal discussions at the University College London circle enriched this research in several ways. I would also like to extend my gratitude to Ms Subashini Shriya and Meenakshi Vashisth for translating some of the difficult Hindi source material. The book has immensely benefitted from my visit to Pakistan. A kind political counsellor, Mr Tariq Karim, at the Pakistan High Commission in New Delhi helped in opening doors to Pakistan for this seemingly harmless academic. My dear friend, Dr Fakhar Bilal provided professional and personal support during this most difficult journey. He opened up his home to me and made this journey the most memorable visit for a third generation 'refugee'. Dr Ali Raza was generous to offer help. I am thankful to authorities in the Punjab Institute of Mental Health, previously the Lahore Mental Hospital. Mr Maqbool Iqbal and Mr Jamshed in particular helped me in finding archival material.

Friends have been the source of joy, hope, love, happiness, and endless discussions and arguments. I am indebted to the support and affection of Arnab, Heeral, Debjani, Radha, Ranjana, Sonia, Suvobrata, Somak, Suparna, Saurabh, Madhuri, Om Lata, and Meenakshi. A special cheer to these friendships and the times that have gone by and to the years that are about to come! These friendships have sustained me through the most difficult times of my life. I have been extremely lucky to have such an intellectually stimulating group of friends.

Finally, I wish to express my deepest gratitude and love to my family. They have been the source of unconditional affection and support. I thank Mami, Mama, and Harshit for their immense support, and Nana and Arun Mama for love and encouragement. I am indebted to Sudha aunty for always standing by me in my academic endeavours, and Tanvi and Tanmay for sprinkling my life with delight, love, and joy. Thank you Masi, Mumma, and Nani. As the saying in Punjabi goes, *Mawa Thandhiya Chahwa*. They have been the coolest shade in the harshest of summers. Finally, I would like to thank my partner Divyanshu for helping me in completing and finalizing the manuscript. His presence has made this intellectual journey more enriching.

Dr Indrani Sen helped me survive both emotionally and intellectually the untimely loss of Dr Biswamoy Pati, who unfortunately could not see this book in the print form. This shall remain one of my deepest regrets. The book took me three years but I kept my promise made to him! I would like to dedicate this book to my dear 'Sir', Dr Biswamoy Pati. He was a father figure, mentor, teacher, and friend.

Introduction

Let us run away to Lahore or Dhaka since they are foreign countries now, but there are asylums there too.[1]

Asrar-ul-Haq Majaz (1911–1955) was admitted to the Ranchi Mental Hospital in the 1950s.[2] When Majaz met Kazi Nazrul Islam (1899–1976) at the same institution, he urged him to run away to Lahore or Dhaka, but he soon realized the futility of the situation as mental hospitals were also found in the newly decolonized nation. The spread of lunatic asylums in the colonies was an imperative consequence of colonialism. Colonialism brought with itself the engines

---

[1] This dialogue appears in the television serial *Kahkashan* (Doordarshan, 1990), in the episode on Asrar-ul-Haq Majaz, with commentary by Ali Sardar Jafri. The TV serial was written and produced by Ali Sardar Jafri.

[2] See Ali Sardar Jafri, *Lucknow ki Panch Rateein* (Delhi: Rajkamal Prakashan, 1998), 56.

of modernity.[3] An important apparatus of colonial modernity was the lunatic asylum. It was later designated in official terminology as the mental hospital.

Asylums in India were established from the latter half of the eighteenth century. The earliest asylum was established in 1745 in Bombay.[4] Lunatic asylums were soon set up in Calcutta and Madras in 1787 and 1794 respectively.[5] The foci of this study are lunatic asylums in two regions, namely the United Provinces (Agra, Benaras, Bareilly, and Lucknow) and the Punjab (Delhi and Lahore) in colonial north India. The book probes the worlds of social histories of medicine and culture as pivotal entry points into what constitutes madness and deviancy in asylum records. It will also be the first one to bring together institutional and non-institutional histories of insanity by focusing on Hindi medical literature. Psychiatric repertoire found its way into the Hindi vernacular wherein the meaning and context differed dramatically. Therefore, the study traces the emergence of 'mind sciences' in Hindi during the period

[3] Historians over the past few decades have questioned the overarching notions about Western modernity and its transportation to colonies. Partha Chatterjee emphasizes the contradictions of colonialism and the difference with which the colonial state applied modernity in colonies. Chatterjee regards this as the rule of colonial difference. Thomas Metcalf has excellently elucidated the ways in which the British justified their rule based on colonial difference. The paraphernalia of colonial modernity had in its bag educational institutions (schools, colleges, and universities) and medical institutions (hospitals, dispensaries, and asylums). The first work to emphasize colonial difference in somewhat different terms was Frantz Fanon's *Black Skin, White Masks*, translated by Charles Lam Markmann (London: Pluto Press, 2008 [first published in French in 1952]). For further reference, see Ashis Nandy, *The Intimate Enemy: Loss and Recovery of Self Under Colonialism* (Delhi: Oxford University Press, 1983); Partha Chatterjee, *The Nation and Its Fragments: Colonial and Postcolonial Histories* (Princeton: Princeton University Press, 1993); Thomas R. Metcalf, *Ideologies of the Raj* (Cambridge: Cambridge University Press, 1995); Dipesh Chakrabarty, *Provincializing Europe: Postcolonial Thought and Historical Difference* (Princeton: Princeton University Press, 2000).

[4] D. G. Crawford, *A History of the Indian Medical Service 1600–1913*, vol. 2 (London: Thacker & Co., 1914), 400.

[5] Crawford, *A History of the Indian Medical Service 1600–1913*, vol. 2, 415, 429.

of high nationalism. The book unmasks the irrationalities of colonialism and nationalism by contextualizing the social, cultural, and political frames in which racial, primordial, psychical, spiritual, and psychiatric understanding of madness were enmeshed, resulting in a peculiar milieu.

The nineteenth century saw the spread of lunatic asylums all over the world. Roy Porter argues that the 'asylums became a panacea; it was the nineteenth century which brought a skyrocketing in the number and scale of mental hospitals. In England, patient numbers climbed from perhaps 10,000 in 1800 to ten times that number in 1900'.[6] The birth of modern psychiatry has been traced to the moment when Philippe Pinel stroked the chains off of the insane at Saltpetre. This representative moment is believed to have changed the course of how we understand madness and its cure. Nonetheless, madness was fettered in the rhetoric of the moral management system. This system propagated the idea about management of madness through kindness and observation. The superintendent of a lunatic asylum was regarded as a father figure who was supposed to use kindness and control to bring back those individuals whose mind had gone astray. This moral management was based on the principle of self-control, which, added with the right amount of sedatives, purgatives, and medicines, was the key to cure insanity. In spite of this initial enthusiasm, the turn of century events led to disillusionment as the number of 'incurables' continued to increase. This forced psychiatrists, who by then had a separate professional identity, to understand the disease in more biological terms. The consequences were far-reaching. An array of intrusive and inventive technologies was developed, such as electroconvulsive therapy (ECT) and lobotomy. It was also an era when psychotropic drugs started to be manufactured and consumed on a massive scale.

The confinement of madness within four walls has been an issue of intense debate. The pioneering argument offered by Michel Foucault in *Madness and Civilization* led to a spurt in research on the history of psychiatry, then a marginal area of study. For Foucault, madness was a construct that took place in the period c.1500–1800. He asserted that 'we must try to return, in history, to that zero point in the course

⁶ Roy Porter, *Madness: A Brief History* (Oxford: Oxford University Press, 2002), 112.

of madness at which madness is an undifferentiated experience, a not yet divided experience of division itself'.[7] For Foucault, there existed in history a dialogue between reason and unreason. The madman was an ambiguous figure who fascinated and scared the world of Renaissance. The mad person was condemned and confined on a large scale during the period. The establishment of the Hopital General in France supposedly heralded the victory of reason. In the seventeenth century, enormous houses of confinement were built that were peopled by the mad, the unemployed, and the poor debauched. As Foucault points out, 'one out of every hundred inhabitants of the city of Paris were confined'.[8] The 'great confinement' became a norm in all European countries. Foucault argues that madness or deviance in any given society depends on the manner in which it is defined by the elite. These privileged few employ power and knowledge in order to invent the 'abnormal'.

Historians of colonial psychiatry have conceded that there was no 'great confinement' in colonies. The colonial state displayed an anxiety, bordering almost on psychosis, as far as its relationship with the colonized was concerned and in this context the investigation of psychiatric power assumes significance. The present book unravels various facets of psychiatry during the colonial period. The focus is on government policies, legal processes, diagnosis and treatment, the everyday behind the walls, and individual case histories. Earlier works on this area have ignored the role of law. This study focuses on important legislation related to lunacy. It seeks to bring to the fore regional specificities. It questions Waltraud Ernst's argument that by early twentieth century, psychiatrists in colonial India were practising 'modern' psychiatry.[9]

---

[7] Michel Foucault, *Madness and Civilization: A History of Insanity in the Age of Reason*, translated by Richard Howard (London: Routledge, 2001), xi.

[8] Foucault, *Madness and Civilization*, 42.

[9] Waltraud Ernst, 'Crossing the Boundaries of "Colonial Psychiatry": Reflections on the Development of Psychiatry in British India, c. 1870–1940', *Culture, Medicine and Psychiatry*, vol. 35, no. 4 (December 2011): 537. Also see Waltraud Ernst, *Colonialism and Transnational Psychiatry: The Development of an Indian Mental Hospital in British India, c. 1920–1940* (London: Anthem Press, 2013).

My main argument is that psychiatry was fettered by colonialism at least in the two regions of the United Provinces and the Punjab.

The focus of psychiatry was on those groups and individuals that could not be brought into the fold of the law. The policies related to handling lunacy attempted to bring irascible individuals and groups under political control. 'Madness' as a term encompassed various forms of deviancies ranging from vagrancy to spirit drinking to hemp drug users. These types of behaviour were considered dangerous and thus were shut away in the asylums. J. C. Penny, the superintendent of the Delhi Asylum, wrote:

> I notice that there have been persons who, intoxicated by bhang, became uproarious, and who were no doubt very violent and perhaps dangerous at the time. But are they fit persons for detention in a asylum, or are they not rather moral offenders and amenable to the law? That there is a form of insanity consequent on excessive use of intoxicating drugs we know too well, but the cases I refer to are not such. They are perfectly rational and intelligent and well aware of the causes of their being sent as 'pagles'. I may be wrong in my view, and the inebriate, say a soldier, dhobie or maither [mehtars], who gets violent from bhang, is one who should be in asylum, and kept there till he is cured of his habit.[10]

The harmless and the incurable insane were on the other hand left on the streets. This work does not deny the existence of mental illnesses, rather it questions the exigencies of colonial governance that prioritized the 'bad' over and above the 'mad'. Madness and delinquency were, thus, coterminous with each other. The asylums thus played a significant role in colonial governance. This case-specific study of the six asylums in north India also allows us to understand how Indians used the psychiatric services for their benefit. It is pertinent to note that the colonial institutional infrastructure formed the basis of psychiatry in the postcolonial period.

New sites such as Akolah in Hyderabad district and Fyzabad were considered to be suitable for the establishment of asylums in the North

---

[10] The Annual Report of the Lunatic Asylums in the Punjab for the year 1875, the National Archives of India (hereafter, NAI).

Western Provinces.[11] Kanpur and Meerut were also considered as feasible sites. It was found expedient to construct an asylum at Raipur for the lunatics of the Chhattisgarh division.[12] For Punjab it was planned to have one near Peshawar and another close to Multan.[13] An asylum was also proposed to be established at Larkana for the Bombay Presidency. The proposals were based on a rough computation of the insane in the respective areas. While proposing new asylums for the Bombay Presidency Dr Arnott, inspector general of the Indian Medical Department, noted:

> It is believed that the population of the presidency of Bombay and its Dependencies is about 15 million. If, then, the computation that there is one lunatic in every thousand of population is correct, it may be easily calculated how many there are in the Bombay presidency, and how inadequate the accommodation is ... there can be no doubt there are very many who might be advantageously confined, instead of being allowed to range about.[14]

This discussion would indicate that there was considerable debate among the officials on the issue of multiplication of the lunatic asylums, and that the British Indian government was keen to establish new structures where 'mad' people could be contained. In reality, however, all this was merely rhetoric. The debate remained only at the level of discussion and nothing much was done to increase the number of asylums. No asylums came up at any of the places mentioned earlier. Moreover, at the

[11] Letters from J. G. Cordery, Assistant Resident at Hyderabad, to E. C. Bayley, Secretary to the Government of India, and Letter from Major L. F. Andrew, Officiating Secretary to the Chief Commissioner of Oude, to E. C. Bayley, Secretary to the Government, Home Dept. Proceedings/Public Branch, 23 January 1869, NAI.

[12] Letters from J. G. Cordery to E. C. Bayley, and Letter from Major L. F. Andrew to E. C. Bayley. Proceedings/Public Branch, 23 January 1869, NAI.

[13] E. C. Bayley, Secretary to the Government of India, cites an extract from the Governor General in Council, 2 October 1867, Home Dept. Proceedings, October 1867, NAI.

[14] Provision of Lunatic Asylums in India, Home Dept./Public Branch, File No. 172–174, 23 January 1869, NAI.

beginning of the twentieth century, existing asylums were amalgamated and centralized. This step was related to the cost reduction policies of the colonial state. The colonial policies were based on the principle of economizing the mental health care system. The book argues that while large-scale establishments were instituted, the basic ideal was that of doing the 'bare minimum'.

Another reason as to why asylums were not localized or multiplied was that a proportion of lunatics was incarcerated in prisons. In 1889 information regarding the non-criminal lunatics in the jails was sought by the government, which enquired, 'Where are the non-criminal lunatics kept in jail for observation, and under what orders?'[15] These lunatics were kept under observation before being sent to the lunatic asylums. Most of them were 'supposed' lunatics, an important category that itself invites explanation. Act XVIII of 1886 amended Act XXXVI of 1858 and a clause (6A) was added. According to the clause:

> Where a person is found wandering at large who is deemed to be a lunatic, or where a person believed to be dangerous by the reason of lunacy, is apprehended and sent to the Magistrate or the Commissioner of Police, or where, on report on information that a person deemed to be lunatic ... the Magistrate or the Commissioner of Police, on the request of the medical officer, may be, by order in writing, authorize the detention of the supposed lunatic for such time, not exceeding ten days, as in the opinion of the Magistrate or the Commissioner of Police, may be necessary to enable the medical office to form an opinion on the question whether or not the supposed lunatic is a person with whom a certificate in the form A in the Schedule to this Act ought to be signed.[16]

The Act of 1886 shows the manner in which the colonial state criminalized the insane. It empowered the authorities to detain not only those who were insane but also those whom they thought could be dangerous

---

[15] Proposed Discontinuance of the Practice of Including the Health Statistics of Non-Criminal Lunatics Kept in Jails for Observation in Return of Sickness and Mortality of the Prisoners, Home Dept./Jail Branch, File No. 107 to 109, August 1889, NAI.

[16] Act no. XVIII of 1886, amended Act XXXVI of 1858, Legislative Dept., NAI.

by the reason of lunacy. As a rule these lunatics were to be kept in prison only for a limited period of ten days.

The history of psychiatry in India is underdeveloped. The present study aims to fill the existing gaps. It looks closely at asylums in Agra, Benaras, Bareilly, Lucknow, Delhi, and Lahore in north India. This study covers the period from around the 1800s to 1950. By doing so, it does not simply provide a chronological narrative; rather it attempts to uncover intricate histories of the asylums and 'madness' in colonial north India.[17]

The book also brings to the fore the non-institutional histories of madness. While few ended up in the asylums, most people suffering from insanity were cared for by their families and the local *vaidyas*, *ojhas*, shamans, and pundits. However, Western medicine denigrated indigenous healing traditions forcing them to reconceptualize and reinvent themselves. Practitioners of indigenous medicine felt threatened and made rigorous attempts to modernize their practice. Not only were the Western attacks irrational but the attempts to reform were also absurd. Occurring at the peak of high nationalism, these forms of attacks were often intertwined with puritanical ideas and reflected a narrow vision arising from parochial issues related to caste, class, community, and nation.

Psychiatric diseases, unlike other illnesses, were difficult to diagnose thereby lending power to imperial authorities and later to anticolonial nationalism, which used them to their respective advantages. Confirming whether a person's behaviour suited the racial attitudes or complied with gendered and community rules became the need of the time. Psychiatric categories were engendered and so were their cures, streamlining behaviours of people who crossed their boundaries. For example, faqirs were often declared 'insane' by the colonizers because of their non-conforming way of life. At the same time, the rhetoric that masturbation can result in madness was translated in contemporary Hindi medical literature very differently. Ideas about masturbation, which posed an imminent threat to manhood, were incorporated in the nationalist discourses and was variously interpreted as being related to the loss of physical strength and

---

[17] It may be mentioned here that the year in which India became independent was also the year of the formation of the Indian Psychiatrist Society.

mental ability. On the other hand, hysteria as a category was utilized to streamline gender rules especially related to women who had fallen into the trap of modernity.

The main sources for reconstructing the histories of madness are the annual reports available at the NAI, the Uttar Pradesh State Archives, and the Punjab State Archives. The legislation related to lunacy is an important source for understanding the legal structure of dealing with lunacy that evolved during the nineteenth and twentieth centuries. I have used minutes, enquiries, and commission reports related to lunacy policies to comprehend official policies. Further, official writings and semi-autobiographical accounts of the superintendents of the mental hospitals—such as G. F. W. Ewens' *Insanity in India* (1908), Overbeck-Wright's *Lunacy in India* (1921), and C. J. Lodge Patch's *A Critical Review of the Punjab Mental Hospitals from 1840–1930* (1931)—are at best 'valuable compilations of fact, and at worst, they are old-fashioned, narrowly conceived and somewhat triumphalist volumes celebrating the progress of "European medicine"'.[18] The medical journals of the period such as *The Indian Medical Gazette*, *Lancet*, *British Medical Journal*, and *Journal of Mental Sciences* are other significant source materials. The chapter on non-institutional histories is based on Hindi medical literature. A wide variety of sources such as pamphlets, books, magazines, and articles published in medical journals have been used to construct histories of curing madness in the Hindi vernacular.

My visits to the Agra, Benares, Bareilly, and Lahore mental hospitals have permitted me to gather source materials including the case registers and case notes recovered from the Agra and Lahore Mental Hospitals respectively. These visits have proved critical for investigating the ruptures and continuities between the colonial and postcolonial practices of psychiatry. Psychiatry continues to be a surrogate child of medicine due to its restrictive growth during the colonial period. Many of the mental hospitals are 100 to 150 years old.[19] The stigma of mental illness

---

[18] Shula Marks, 'What Is Colonial about Colonial Medicine? And What Happened to Imperialism and Health?', *Social History of Medicine*, vol. 10, no. 2 (1997): 205.

[19] In July 2013, the Supreme Court of India issued notice to the centre and states concerning the pathetic state of mental hospitals in the country. It was

permeates through the colonial language of 'confinement' and 'control'. The residual past pervades the present of these institutions and *only* the trained eyes of a historian can discern the continuity of the past in the present, or the present in the past. This research brings forth the colonial legacies of contemporary psychiatry.

The study is based upon an interdisciplinary approach with an eye for context-specific detail and wider historiographical currents in writing histories of the 'mad'. Frantz Fanon's insights about the psyche of the colonizer and colonized, Michel Foucault's ideas on the knowledge/power nexus, Edward Said's perspectives on the European 'Self' and the colonized 'Other', and Roy Porter's explorations of the social history of medicine provide essential tools for unravelling the racist and arbitrary attitudes of colonial psychiatry.

The power of psychiatric knowledge in the colonies was questioned by Fanon in a somewhat unique manner, almost a decade before Foucault. Fanon was a psychiatrist by profession. He raised his voice against the prevailing racism in the psychological and psychiatric theories of the period. In his seminal work *Black Skin, White Masks*,[20] Fanon uncovered the ways in which racism was internalized by the colonizer and the colonized. He used psychoanalysis to unmask the perceptions about the self in both 'black' and 'white'. The whites regarded themselves as superior while the blacks considered themselves inferior. For Fanon, colonialism was itself a sort of madness caused by racism. Colonialism ripped apart the identity of the colonized and she/he hated his/her language, culture, and skin colour. Fanon asserted that 'after much reluctance, the scientists had conceded that the Negro was a human being; *in vivo* and *in vitro* the Negro had been proved analogous to the white man: the same morphology, the same histology'.[21] The colonizers regarded themselves as superior, in other words 'superhuman'. The superiority complex had

---

pointed out that some of these mental hospitals were 100 to 150 years old. It was urged that these institutions should be made autonomous and well-trained psychiatrists, neurologists, and mental health workers should be appointed. For further details, see J. Venkatesan, 'SC Issues Notice to States, Centre on Condition of Mental Hospitals', *The Hindu*, 9 July 2013.

20 Fanon, *Black Skin, White Masks*.
21 Fanon, *Black Skin, White Masks*, 90.

stripped them of humanity since they considered themselves far above people of colour. The objectification had an adverse effect on both the colonizer and the colonized.

Megan Vaughan has worked on the history of psychiatry in Africa. She states, 'I was curious as to why colonial administration had felt the need to define and confine the "lunatic". I think I was hoping for the colonial equivalent of what Foucault called the "great confinement", a colonial story of massive institutionalization for the purpose of maintaining social control.'[22] Vaughan, along with other historians, did not find in colonies the 'great confinement' in the Foucauldian sense. Then why did the colonial state feel the need to set up lunatic asylums? Numerous works have tried to address this question. Vaughan suggests that 'the history of Zomba Lunatic Asylum [Nyasaland] and the legislation associated with it reflect the ambiguities, uncertainties and dangers felt by Europeans to be inherent in a situation of their own making, as well as the development of thought on their responsibility for African "welfare"'.[23] According to her, 'if the voices of the "alleged lunatic" are unclear, the records nevertheless often tell us an interesting story. In particular, they reflect on the process by which the magistrate sought to define "mad" behaviour in a group of subjects whose normal behaviour he [magistrate] usually regarded as "alien", to say the least.'[24] In other words, the 'normal' behaviour of 'natives' was often considered 'abnormal'. Richard Keller similarly opined that colonial psychiatrists found even 'ostensibly "normal" North Africans to exhibit a range of pathological behaviors that rendered the general population inherently dangerous to the social order.'[25]

---

[22] Megan Vaughan, *Curing Their Ills: Colonial Power and African Illness* (Stanford: Stanford University Press, 1991), ix.

[23] Megan Vaughan, 'Idioms of Madness: Zomba Lunatic Asylum, Nyasaland, in the Colonial Period', *Journal of Southern African Studies* vol. 9, no. 2 (April 1983): 219.

[24] Vaughan, *Curing Their Ills*, 102.

[25] Richard C. Keller, 'Taking Science to the Colonies: Psychiatric Innovation in France and North Africa', in *Psychiatry and Colonialism*, edited by Sloan Mahone and Megan Vaughan (New York: Palgrave Macmillan, 2007), 25.

Jock McCulloch points out,

> The old racism was concerned with measuring the native's body: the lit-
> erature from the nineteenth and early twentieth centuries is filled with
> attempts to discover a key to the African's backwardness in the size or
> structure of his brain ... modern theories about race have tended to con-
> centrate upon the mentality and sociability of colonial peoples, presuming
> to have found the reason for their backwardness in their personality or
> culture.[26]

Keller argues that 'by the turn of the twentieth century, thinking about
"mind" in an increasingly biological fashion intersected with a new
infatuation with comparative psychology. Social anthropologists, phi-
losophers, and psychiatrists began a nearly obsessive documentation of
the functions of what they called "civilized" or European and "primitive"
mentalities.'[27]

Historians of colonial psychiatry have conceded that there existed a
latent agenda in the practice(s) of colonial psychiatry. This agenda was
related to the needs of governance and control over the 'native' populations. Can it be argued then that colonial psychiatry was all about
control and governance? It would be wrong and reductionist to assume
that psychiatry in colonies was all about management of the 'native'
mind. As stated before, psychiatry in colonies was limited in practice
and that there was never any 'great confinement' as in the West. Mahone
argues that

> psychiatry, or any form of psychological medicine, as a discipline was
> poorly represented in the colonial context in East Africa, but despite the
> lack of institutional support and resources and an inconsistent medical
> agenda on the part of colonial governments, an ad hoc professionalism
> grew out of the small network of East African asylums in Kenya, Uganda,
> Tanganyika and Zanzibar.[28]

---

[26] Jock McCulloch, *Colonial Psychiatry and 'the African Mind'* (Cambridge:
Cambridge University Press, 1995), 5.

[27] Keller, 'Taking Science to the Colonies', 24.

[28] Sloan Mahone, 'East African Psychiatry and the Practical Problems of
Empire', in *Psychiatry and Colonialism*, edited by Sloan Mahone and Megan
Vaughan (New York: Palgrave Macmillan, 2007), 41.

McCulloch observes lunatic asylums, hospitals, dispensaries, lock hospitals, and reformatories offered 'evidence of the civic virtue of settler societies', and supported it by demonstrating the ultimately philanthropic nature of colonialism through symbolic value.[29] Vaughan, in a similar vein, has pointed out that, 'unremarkable in every other way, what was remarkable about the Zomba asylum was its early foundation. This was a time when government expenditure on medical and educational services for African was virtually non-existent [sic]'.[30]

Psychiatry in colonies played a complex role. The colonial asylums emerged as places where the 'bad' and the 'mad' could be incarcerated. These should be situated alongside other institutions of education and medicine that demonstrated the philanthropic and humanitarian side of colonialism. It is in these asylums that eventually the 'science of psychiatry' grew. This science was used by both the colonizer and the colonized. There was never a clear-cut established agenda for psychiatric treatment on the part of the colonial state. Psychiatry along with other disciplines and subdisciplines of medicine and science got enmeshed with the larger project of empire-building. This study will further dwell on these complexities without losing sight of issues related to control and discipline. It will also attempt to demonstrate that psychiatric control had several strands.

Before going further, it is imperative to review the existing historiography on colonial psychiatry in India. Waltraud Ernst[31] and James H. Mills'[32] writings are significant scholarly contributions examining the role of psychiatry in colonial India. Ernst's focus is on the European insane in British India, and the major concern throughout is 'the intersection of race and class in the Raj and the manner in which psychiatrists and administrators employed discrimination to maintain white supremacy in India'.[33] However, Ernst's belief that the number

---

[29] McCulloch, *Colonial Psychiatry and 'the African Mind'*, 43–5.

[30] Vaughan, *Curing Their Ills*, 121.

[31] Waltraud Ernst, *Mad Tales from the Raj: The European Insane in British India, 1800–1858* (London: Routledge, 1991).

[32] James H. Mills, *Madness, Cannabis and Colonialism: The 'Native-Only' Lunatic Asylums of British India, 1857–1900* (Great Britain: Macmillan, 2000).

[33] Waltraud Ernst, 'Madness and Colonial Spaces: British India, c. 1800–1947', in *Madness, Architecture and the Built Environment*, edited by Leslie Topp, James Moran, and Jonathan Andrews (London: Routledge, 2007), 217.

of patients in the asylums in British India was too few leads her to the assessment that 'Western medicine and its emergent offshoot, psychiatry, lent themselves especially well to purposes of ideological legitimating'.[34] Such a view needs to be resituated in the broader context of colonial institutions of medicine and punishment. She has recently shifted her attention to the Ranchi Mental Hospital which was established in the twentieth century.[35] Ernst's claim that psychiatry practised in early twentieth century was 'modern' and 'progressive' is also not entirely convincing. Mills's approach, on the other hand, differs from that of Ernst, as he emphasizes that 'the asylum regime spread only in the post-1857 period'.[36] Another important contribution to the field is Debjani Das's work on the asylums of Bengal. Her work discuses and emphasizes on how the definition and treatment of insanity developed in the asylums of Bengal before the transfer of power occurred from the East India Company to the Crown in 1858.[37] Das states, 'It was in the asylums that definitions of insanity were forged, expanded, modified, corrected, and extended through experiments on the inmates of the asylums.'[38]

Mills argues that the treatment regimes established in this period were 'a combination of moral management programmes and drug therapy aimed at subduing and resting the patient before putting them to work'.[39] Words such as 'reform' and 'subduing' exaggerate the intended aims of lunatic asylums. The asylum policy was based more on indifference, neglect, and discipline. Therefore, these institutions cannot be regarded as mere instruments of brute force. The asylums were failed attempts of bringing modernity to colonies as part of the emerging modern

---

[34] Waltraud Ernst, 'Idioms of Madness and Colonial Boundaries: The Case of the European and "Native" Mentally Ill in Early Nineteenth-Century British India', *Comparative Studies in Society and History*, vol. 39, no. 1 (1997): 169.

[35] Ernst, 'Crossing the Boundaries of "Colonial Psychiatry"': 544.

[36] James H. Mills, 'The History of Modern Psychiatry in India, 1858–1957', *History of Psychiatry*, vol. 12, no. 4 (2001): 433–4.

[37] Debjani Das, *Houses of Madness: Insanity and Asylums of Bengal in Nineteenth-Century India* (New Delhi, Oxford University Press, 2015), 9.

[38] Das, *Houses of* Madness, 9.

[39] Mills, 'The History of Modern Psychiatry in India', 444.

medical sciences. The book explicates the policy of colonial indifference towards the mentally ill and mental illness at large. Asylums by their very origin were part of the disciplinary regimes which found catalysts in the colonial milieu making them more prone to quotidian violence, neglect, and control. This research shows that by the late colonial period psychiatry became a negligent part of the medical sciences. The early fervour was over and it was a group of psychiatrists that was able to give any definitive shape to psychiatry in India. The state consciously backed off from any sort of structural support leaving psychiatry fettered and underdeveloped.

Amit Ranjan Basu provides the only extant scholarly contribution connecting vernacular medical literature and the emergence of psychiatry in nineteenth- and twentieth-century Bengal. Through a study of Bengali periodicals he analyses the ways in which some of the Western ideas were internalized. Basu points out that 'there existed a trend that Bengali narratives on psychiatry mainly translated English articles and documented clinically observed cases of various disorders.'[40] In the context of the politics of princely India, Shruti Kapila analyses the case histories of Shivaji IV of Kolhapur and Mir Faiz Mohhammad Khan of the Sind state of Khairpurto to highlight how insanity and 'unmanliness' crossed the well-guarded norms of princely personhood.[41] Nile Green analyses the annual reports of the asylums and remarks that 'the population of beggars, mendicants, faqirs and pauper gradually rose by the end of nineteenth century. What these data demonstrate is the use of the asylum in a colonial anti-vagrant policy of clearing the streets of "insane" mendicants.'[42] The works of Green and Kapila probe deeper into the lives of those alleged to be 'insane'; these studies are welcome contributions as they direct our attention to the need to study case histories of

---

[40] Amit Ranjan Basu, 'Emergence of a Marginal Science in a Colonial City: Reading Psychiatry in Bengali Periodicals', *Indian Economic and Social History Review*, vol. 41, no. 2 (2004): 119–20.

[41] Shruti Kapila, 'Masculinity and Madness: Princely Personhood and Colonial Sciences of Mind in Western India, 1871–1940', *Past and Present*, vol. 187, no. 1 (May 2005): 130, 144–5.

[42] Nile Green, 'Jack Sepoys and the Dervishes: Islam and the Indian Soldier in Princely India', *Journal of Royal Asiatic Society*, vol. 18, no. 1 (2008): 39.

individual patients. Basu's work on the other hand, looks at the penetration of prevalent psychiatric discourses in Bengali texts. This work extends and elaborates historiography in several ways. It opens up Hindi medical literature to historians of psychiatry in India. Case studies of individual patients have been used here as a new genre of writing the social history of medicine.

The present book is divided into five chapters. Chapter 1 begins by describing the salient features of the Lunacy Act of 1858. The Act contained provisions for the maintenance and care of the 'native' insane in colonial India. This chapter also examines the role of enquiries such as that of James Clark and the Indian Hemp Drugs Commission (IHDC). It suggests that the language of reform was crucial since it justified the existence of the lunatic asylums and projected the humanitarian side of the Raj. Nonetheless, the criminalization of the insane continued throughout the nineteenth century. The processes of medicalization and professionalization were pushed forward due to the IHDC's investigation into the relationship of hemp use with insanity. The Commission unveiled the defective character of the lunatic asylums. The members of the Commission exposed the malpractices and demanded centralization. By the beginning of the twentieth century small asylums were amalgamated into larger ones. This centralization triggered the professionalization of psychiatry during the first half of the twentieth century. The lunatic asylums were re-named as mental hospitals. The twentieth century was a period of flux in the history of psychiatry in India. The 1912 Act was a significant attempt to consolidate lunacy laws. This period also witnessed changes due to individual efforts. These individuals were usually superintendents of the central asylums.

The second chapter delineates the structures of the colonial lunatic asylums. It throws light on the ways in which madness was managed behind the walls of the asylums. The chapter looks at the role architecture played in the organization of insanity. It also throws light on the hierarchies that existed among the medical staff, and the manner in which these hierarchies actually played out in terms of staff–patient relationships. The diagnosis and classification reveal the latent attitudes of psychiatry in colonial north India. Treatment and medicinal practices have also been elaborated in detail.

Chapter 3 looks at everyday life in the asylums. The routine activities such as 'employment and amusement,' 'diet and medicine', and 'reform and reward' are the foci of the chapter. An attempt is made to understand how the banal lives of the inmates were organized. The 'trope of mundane' allows us to focus on the nebulous evidences of the connections between the effort to enforce discipline on the life of inmates and the problems related to the working of the colonial asylums. Asylums played a medico-punitive role throughout colonial India. The everyday patterns of domination, adjustment, and resistance allowed the reconstruction of the social lives of the inmates.

The fourth chapter examines a few case histories. These histories have been retreived from diverse sources which include asylum case registers, annual reports, official files, journal articles, and monographs written by the superintendents of the mental hospitals. This chapter tries to shed light on who these patients really were. It not only throws light on their socio-economic background, but through these records the chapter helps one comprehend the manner in which the patient's insanity was understood and constructed through medical case books. The chapter focuses on the interplay of insanity, individuals (including families in some cases), and the institutions.

The final chapter delineates madness outside the asylums. *Unmada* or severe psychiatric condition in Ayurveda was understood as originating due to the imbalances of three basic *dosas* or elements. The circulation of Western medical knowledge and ideas led to the reshaping of the basic concepts of mental illness. This chapter reveals how insanity and its cures were reconceptualized in Hindi medical literature. The Western and the Eastern notions of the mind/body dichotomy were integrated. It also delves into certain psychosexual pathologies that emerged during the period. Nationalistic medical acquisitions of psychiatric diseases often reflect gender bias, communal hostilities, and fears of degeneration. The bodies of the Self/Other were reformulated in the discourses of mental illnesses. The chapter examines select books, magazines, and literature in Hindi that re-imagined the meaning of psychiatric illness and its cures.

The state was apathetic towards the mentally ill. Harmless lunatics were considered to be burdensome and the practice of incarcerating them was discouraged. The 'troublesome' and the 'unruly' were considered fit to be sent to the asylum whereas the harmless were left to the care of the families. The jail continued for long to be the place to incarcerate the 'mad'. While psychiatry remained 'marginal' throughout the period of our study, its power was imminently used in suppressing and streamlining 'problematic' elements of society. This is not to argue that people did not receive any benefit from these institutions. The book will show that the lower classes turned the logic of colonialism upside down and sometimes used these institutions as a 'refuge' for themselves and their relatives. The walls of these asylums were permeable and asylum structures evolved and devolved over the longer period of colonialism. However, colonialism, which itself was based on exploitation, violence, and racial ideology, passed these characteristics to all its central and marginal institutions. These ideas pervaded through the writings of 'enlightened psychiatrists' who demeaned Indian traditional practices regarding madness and its cure. This thereby created a wide cleavage between the Eastern and Western knowledge systems, which is still palpable to the present day.

1 Lunacy and the Colonial State

The government, by a warrant which shall set forth the ground of belief that such prisoner is of unsound mind, may order the removal of such person to a lunatic asylum, or other fit place of safe custody. [1]

This chapter maps the history of psychiatry in India. It examines the variegated processes of professionalization, modernization, and Indianization along with the obstacles that colonialism created in their paths. These processes, which began at the turn of the twentieth century, were far from complete even on the eve of Independence. The chapter argues that psychiatry remained at the margins of medicine as the colonial state maintained an indifferent attitude towards the development of the mental sciences.

Highlighting contributions of individual psychiatrists and juxtaposing them with those of the colonial state, the chapter locates psychiatrists as

[1] Act no. IV of 1849, An Act for the Safe Custody of Criminal Lunatics, 1849, NAI.

historical actors at the centre of the history of colonial psychiatry during the period. Historians working on lunatic asylums have rightly pointed out that there was no 'great confinement' in the colonies.[2] However, the empire of asylums in India saw a definite growth, and official debates over the nature and administration of them flourished within the official circles. The chapter delineates the macro-histories of the official persons and policies of and policing by colonial psychiatry in India.

Legal Insanity

Asylums marched along with colonialism in India. Much before the consolidation of imperial power, the incarceration of the insane became a widespread phenomenon. The insane hospitals were initially opened for the sequestration of insane soldiers but soon the provision was extended to the 'native' insanes. In 1800, an abstract from the Secretary to the Governor General in Council authorized 'the reception of the insane natives of various descriptions not in the company's service into the same house with the insane native soldiers for whose reception the hospital at Mongyr was originally established'.[3] The histories of the establishment of the lunatic asylums are not uniform. The asylums grew in number along with the expansion of the empire. By 1802, the Governor in Council ordered the establishment of five lunatic asylums in the Bengal presidency.

Writing in 1827, Scottish physician Andrew Halliday provided a general survey of the six lunatic asylums functioning at the time in

[2] Waltraud Ernst, 'The European Insane in British India, 1800–1858: A Case Study in Psychiatry and Colonial Rule', in *Imperial Medicine and Indigenous Societies*, edited by David Arnold (Manchester: Manchester University Press, 1988), 28; Waltraud Ernst, *Mad Tales from the Raj: Colonial Psychiatry in South Asia, 1800–1858* (London: Anthem Press, 2010), 40; Megan Vaughan, *Curing Their Ills: Colonial Power and African Illness* (Palo Alto: Stanford University Press, 1991), ix; Harriet Deacon, 'Robben Island Lunatic Asylum, South Africa, 1846–1910', in *The Confinement of Insane: International Perspectives 1800–1965*, edited by Roy Porter and David Wright (Cambridge, Cambridge University Press, 2003), 51.

[3] Extract from the proceedings of the Board in the Military Department, O.C., no. 23, 6 November 1800, NAI.

the Bengal Presidency.[4] By the 1830s a few more asylums were established. James H. Mills argues that after 1859 there began two decades of unprecedented activity of providing buildings to contain those the British encountered as 'mad' in the Indian population.[5] Waltraud Ernst highlights,

> The creation of Courts of Law, the establishment of police forces and the erection of jails were vital means of guaranteeing English power and of controlling public life. So were other, less conspicuous measures of social control, such as the erection of public hospitals—characteristically called 'police or pauper hospitals'—dispensaries, licensed brothels, workhouses, and last but not least lunatic asylums.[6]

Ernst, though cautious of the concept of social control, argues that it is 'taken up merely as a heuristic device to describe the process'.[7] Such a view fails to situate asylums in the broader context of colonial institutions of medicine and punishment. Asylums and psychiatric knowledge should be considered critically important in the colonial settings. Lunatic asylums were established for twin purposes. The primary reason was to safeguard the public from the 'dangerous' insane and the second rationale was to provide shelter to 'the most unhappy class of human beings'. Thus, asylums were made for both coercive and therapeutic purposes. Existing scholarship has ignored the significant role of law in regulating and managing 'insanity'.[8] Legal frameworks reflect necessities of colonialism

---

[4] Andrew Halliday, *A General View of the Present State of Lunatics and Lunatic Asylums in Great Britain and Ireland and in Some Other Kingdoms* (London: Thomas and George Underwood, 1827), 65.

[5] Mills, *Madness, Cannabis and Colonialism*, 12.

[6] Waltraud Ernst, 'The Establishment of "Native Lunatic Asylums" in Early Nineteenth-Century British India', in *Studies on Indian Medical History*, edited by G. Jan Meulendbeld and Dominik Wujastyk (New Delhi: Motilal Banarasidass, 2001), 155.

[7] Ernst, 'The Establishment of "Native Lunatic Asylums"', 155.

[8] Waltraud Ernst and James H. Mills in their scholarly works have discussed the 1858 Act. The subsequent amendments of the 1858 Act and the 1912 Act have been overlooked. My endeavour would be to contextualize the significant amendments. This chapter tries to unravel the ways in which laws were used

which in turn mirror blurred ideas on governance, benevolence, and social control. The investigation into lunacy laws will help in contextualizing imperatives of psychiatry and colonialism.

In England, by the prerogative of the Crown, the property of the natural born 'idiot' and of those lunatics whose lunacy had been established was delegated to the Lord Chancellor. The Crown regarded this prerogative as *parens patriae* (the ruling monarch who would act as a legal guardian). The care of the lunatic was then assigned to a 'committee of the person', and of his property to a 'committee of the estate'.[9] The order of the law was property-driven rather than person-oriented, and in practice, was usually reserved for cases where control over the family wealth was at issue.[10] In other words, regulation of insanity was closely linked to control over property. In India the general law of England was implemented. According to this law, the care, both of the person and of the property of the lunatic, was being vested in the Crown by virtue of its prerogative.[11] By the charter of 1773, the Crown delegated the responsibilities to the Supreme Court 'to appoint guardians and keepers of the persons and estates of persons deprived of their understanding or reason, and to enquire, hear and determine concerning the same'.[12]

A specific legislative measure related to lunacy in India was introduced by the colonial government only in the mid-nineteenth century. In 1849, an Act for the safe custody of criminal lunatics was passed. Clause VI of the Act states:

> Whereas it shall appear to the government that any person, imprisoned by the sentence of any court, is of unsound mind, the government, by a warrant which shall set forth the ground of belief that such prisoner is of

---

by 'natives' and the colonial state. The legal case histories would help in understanding the nebulous connections between law and medicine.

[9] Clive Unsworth, 'Law and Lunacy in Psychiatry's "Golden Age"', *Oxford Journal of Legal Studies*, vol. 13, no. 4 (1993): 490.

[10] Unsworth, 'Law and Lunacy': 490.

[11] Opinion of the Advocate General, the papers related to the Lunacy Acts No. XXXIV, XXXV and XXXVI of 1858, NAI.

[12] Opinion of the Advocate General, the papers related to the Lunacy Acts No. XXXIV, XXXV and XXXVI of 1858, NAI.

unsound mind, may order the removal of such person to a lunatic asylum, or other fit place of safe custody, there to be kept and treated as the
government shall order; and when it shall appear to the government that
such prisoner has become of sound mind, the government, by a warrant
directed to the person having charged of him, shall remand such prisoner
to the prison from which he was removed, if then still liable to be kept
in custody, or if not, shall order him to be discharged out of custody.[13]

The 1849 Act was extremely significant as it set forth the definition of
legal insanity in India. This Act, based on English law, made the insanity defence possible in India. The discourses of legalism and medicalism
were brought together for the first time in order to define insanity and
their responsibilities related to it.

The reasons for introducing the Act for the safe custody of criminal
lunatics were complex. The first and foremost aim was to provide safety
to the public from the criminal lunatic. The criminal mad person was
feared the most. The Act guaranteed the safety of the public from the
lunatic. Second, the Act demonstrated the philanthropic liberality of
English law to the most unfortunate humans. Psychiatry can indeed be
seen as one of the measures of the 'civilizing' process. Third, it allowed
the safe incarceration of a lunatic away from sight of the public. Ernst
argues that the Act allowed confinement of military servants who
shammed madness when tired of their military duty. She asserts that
'given the insalubrious aspects of military life, lunacy appealed to quite
a few as an alternative to the madness of the service in the East. Not
only simple soldiers … officers, too, sometimes made the most of the
law's insanity clause'.[14] Drinkwater Bethune, the president of the Indian
Law Commission was not in favour of passing the Act. He regarded its
practical application 'far from being in clear and satisfactory state'.[15] In
spite of this initial hesitation, the Act was introduced in India.[16]

The Act became the basis of what is popularly known as the 'insanity plea'. It is difficult to say to what extent the Act provided any relief

[13] Act no. IV of 1849, An Act for the Safe Custody of Criminal Lunatics,
1849, NAI.

[14] Ernst, *Mad Tales from the Raj*, 47–8.

[15] Ernst, *Mad Tales from the Raj*, 48.

[16] Ernst, *Mad Tales from the Raj*, 48.

to Indian subjects. Colonial officials had a stereotyped image related to 'eccentricity of conduct in natives'.[17] This stereotyping should not be ignored while understanding the use of the insanity plea. Norman Chevers's incisive study, *A Manual of Medical Jurisprudence*, delves into the subject of insanity among 'natives'. He discusses in detail methods of judging the insanity or sanity of 'natives':

> Upon committing an act of frantic violence, a native of this country, having undergone examination at the thannah and at the Magistrate's court, is generally placed as soon as possible, in the jail under the observation of the Civil Surgeon. Here it, of course, becomes the duty of the latter at once to endeavour to distinguish how much of any disorder of the intellectual facilities which the culprit may present is dependent on *physical*, and how much on *mental* causes ... the Medical officer may, upon observing that his eyes are inflamed, his head hot, his tongue foul, and his pulse excited, and, upon learning that he is sleepless at night, feel disposed to exercise the remedial portion of his art, and to prescribe purgatives, nauseates, sedatives, low diet and cold affusion ... it is always safer and fairer towards the subject of our scrutiny to leave his case untreated—under the most careful watching ... under these circumstances, it may fairly be expected that the effect of intoxication, whether by *sharab* or *gunja*, will gradually pass off ... and true mania will probably remain unaffected, except in character and degree ... it is only *after the Trial* that the physician can be justified in *treating* the criminal lunatic.[18]

Observation was the key to judgement with regard to lunacy. The vital question, however, here was, to what extent was a fair and a balanced judgement possible in the context of insanity among 'natives'. Chevers's *A Manual of Medical Jurisprudence* reveals an innate bias present in the opinion of the colonizers. The basic characteristics of Indians including caste organization, religion, and customs were regarded as 'abnormal'. This abnormality was measured in terms of the difference between their own and the 'native's' way of life.

Historians working on law and colonialism have shown how laws were tailored to accomplish the needs of colonialism. Bernard Cohn

[17] Norman Chevers, *A Manual of Medical Jurisprudence for Bengal and North-Western Provinces* (Calcutta: Military Orphan Press, 1856).
[18] Chevers, *A Manual of Medical Jurisprudence*, 559–61.

argues that 'the indigenous laws were integrated in a way that had to take into account British ideas of proper discipline, forms of deference, and demeanor that should mark the relations between rulers and ruled'.[19] Radhika Singha locates law as 'the strategic imperative, the search for defensible frontier, which provided one explanation for the dynamic of imperial expansion'.[20] Elizabeth Kolsky, in her recent study, highlights how the process of codification allowed colonial administrators to control unruly British citizens and colonized Indian subjects.[21] She states that 'so great and intricately interlinked were the efforts of codification that British India's most prolific codifier James Fitzjames Stephen was invited by the Parliament to bring his Indian experience to bear upon the ongoing efforts to codify the English law'.[22] In other words, the Indian colony was viewed as an exemplary model of codification by the colonizers. This might be true for the other sets of laws such as the criminal code but as far the lunacy laws were concerned, they were more or less British in form and content. In the absence of any set of clear rules or laws related to lunacy in medieval India, the British were free to transport their own laws. As Cohn observes, 'The laws of these colonies were the laws of Great Britain.'[23] Indian lunacy laws were heavily influenced by, if not an exact replica of, the English lunacy law.

After the passing of the 1849 Act, the next piece of legislation related to lunacy in India was enacted in 1858. Historians working on the history of psychiatry in India have emphasized that the explicit aim of the 1858 Act was to bring 'the legal situation in India in line with that of Britain.'[24] However, mention might be made of an incident that occurred in 1856 which pushed the government to pass this historic Act. The

[19] Bernard Cohn, *Colonialism and Its Forms of Knowledge*, in *The Bernard Cohn Omnibus* (New Delhi: Oxford University Press, 2008), 61.

[20] Radhika Singha, *A Despotism of Law: Crime and Justice in Early Colonial India* (New Delhi: Oxford University Press, 2000), xv.

[21] Elizabeth Kolsky, *Colonial Justice in British India* (New Delhi, Cambridge University Press, 2010), 11.

[22] Elizabeth Kolsky, 'Codification and the Rule of Colonial Difference: Criminal Procedure in British India', *Law and History Review*, vol. 23, no. 3 (2005): 63.

[23] Cohn, *Colonialism and Its Forms of Knowledge*, 57.

[24] Ernst, *Mad Tales from the Raj*, 45.

Superintendent of Bhowanipore and Dullunda Asylums, T. Cantor, wrote to the secretary of the medical board:

> I avail myself of the present occasion to call the attention of the Board to the fact that no Act exists, legalizing, in this Presidency, the admission and detention for treatment in asylums of insane patients. A few days after the asylum had become the property of Government, an instance occurred in which a certain attorney thought proper to discredit my declaration that an insane patient had been discharged to the care of his relations. I was compelled before the Supreme Court to make an affidavit to that effect, and I have been advised that the accidental discharge, only, of the lunatic saved me from legal prosecution. Under such circumstances I am compelled to solicit the Board to obtain protection for my office.[25]

Cantor had handed over William Knox, an inmate of the Bhowanipore Lunatic Asylum, to the latter's daughter, who undertook to take proper care of him. Following the release of Knox, probably within a day or so, Cantor received a letter from Mr T. Sherrington, an attorney:

> I am instructed by a friend of Mr. Knox to make an application to the Supreme Court for his release, he being considered by his friends sufficiently sane to be at liberty and manage the affairs; but previous to taking any measures, I think it is right to enquire of you upon whose authority Mr. Knox was committed to your charge, and under what circumstances and by whom is he detained at the asylum. I will feel obliged by being furnished with this information.[26]

Cantor was forced to supply an affidavit certifying that the government of Bengal instructed him to take care of Knox. Cantor felt threatened and demanded legislative immunity. What is worth noting is that it was the absence of relevant legislation that concerned the officials and not the welfare of the subjects. This incident, though minor in nature, led to

---

[25] Superintendent of Bhowanipore and Dullunda Lunatic Asylums to the Secretary to the Medical Board, 21 February 1857, cited in the papers related to the Lunacy Acts No. XXXIV, XXXV and XXXVI of 1858, NAI.

[26] From T. Sherrington, Attorney at Law, to the Superintendent of the Bhowanipore Lunatic Asylum, 8 January 1856, cited in the papers related to the Lunacy Acts No. XXXIV, XXXV and XXXVI of 1858, NAI.

an extensive debate in official circles. The papers relating to Lunacy Act nos XXXIV, XXXV, and XXXVI found in the NAI give us an insight into the debate that took place in the official circles before the passing of the 1858 Act.

The opinion of the Advocate General was invited on the matter. W. Ritchie, the Advocate General, argued that 'a law was not of an absolute necessity in the way the superintendent of the Bhowanipore Asylum had argued'.[27] Nevertheless, he was of the view that

> it was easy to convince the Supreme Court in the case of Mr. Knox as his lunacy was established, but in cases where lunacy was of subtle nature and one would need the protection of the law [sic]. Giving a background to the general law of lunacy that had existed in India established by the charter of 1773, the crown delegated the responsibilities of a propertied lunatic to the Supreme Court, a reform in the respect is loudly called for.[28]

He felt that recent improvements in English lunacy laws should be brought to India. Ritchie was fixated on the propertied lunatic and management of his/her estate since he averred that 'in order to obtain the protection of the Court for the person or property of a lunatic, a heavy expense (the very lower being, I understand, fifteen hundred Rupees, and varying from that to three thousand Rupees) must be incurred. Unless, therefore, the lunatic has considerable property, recourse to a court is idle'.[29] It is here that he vociferously demanded a reform. It is in a minor paragraph that Ritchie discussed the necessity of proper provision for the pauper lunatics in India.[30]

The Indian Lunacy Act of 1858, though modelled on the English Lunacy Act of 1853, evaded the issue of pauper lunacy. In England the question of pauper lunacy had come to the fore in the period and the

---

[27] Opinion of the Advocate General, the papers related to the Lunacy Acts No. XXXIV, XXXV and XXXVI of 1858, para. 2, NAI.

[28] Opinion of the Advocate General, the papers related to the Lunacy Acts No. XXXIV, XXXV and XXXVI of 1858, para. 2, NAI.

[29] Opinion of the Advocate General, the papers related to the Lunacy Acts No. XXXIV, XXXV and XXXVI of 1858, para. 2, NAI.

[30] Opinion of the Advocate General, the papers related to the Lunacy Acts No. XXXIV, XXXV and XXXVI of 1858, para. 2, NAI.

Lunatics Act of 1845 led to the establishment of a permanent National Lunacy Commission in England. The Act made compulsory the setting up of county and borough asylums to house pauper lunatics.[31] The Lunacy Act of 1853 provided for framing of rules related to pauper lunacy and its management. Issues such as how funds could be raised for providing asylums and how expenses for maintenance of lunatics could be met were addressed by the 1853 Act. In England poverty was officially recognized as a problem to be dealt with, but it was not acknowledged as such in the colonies. Early moderate nationalists blamed the colonial state for the creation of widespread poverty in India. What is evident is the fact that the colonial government was washing its hands off any sort of poor relief. The government officials kept on repeating that only 'dangerous' lunatics and 'harmless' incurables should be kept in the asylums. The Inspector General of Prisons for the North Western Provinces wrote to the government in this context that 'the government cannot undertake to provide for all lunatics nor even for all pauper lunatics'.[32] David Arnold has looked at the issue of poverty and state-sponsored poor relief in colonial India. He remarks that 'the 1837–1838 North Indian famine saw a widespread use of such terms as *paupers*, *vagrants* and the *able bodied* and *deserving poor* that echo poor law legislation in Britain. But despite this rhetoric, there was extreme reticence about adopting similar measures in India'.[33] This reticence was due to the fact that Indians were regarded as being numerically too many to be given systematic state relief. Arnold notes that 'private charity was organized to fill the void by the paucity of state relief but in novel forms of provincial and all-India funds'.[34] He states that 'while

---

[31] Andrew Scull, *The Most Solitary of Afflictions: Madness and Society in Britain, 1700–1900* (New Haven and London: Yale University Press, 1993), 16.

[32] Letter from the Inspector General of Prison of the N. W. Province to the Secretary of the Government of the N. W. Provinces, Proposal for the Construction for the Lunatic Asylum at Agra, Home Dept./Public Branch, File No. 26 to 30, 20 October 1862, NAI.

[33] David Arnold, 'Vagrant India: Famine, Poverty and Welfare under Colonial Rule', in *Cast Out: Vagrancy and Homelessness in Global and Historical Perspective*, edited by A. L. Beier and Paul Ocobock (Ohio: Ohio University Press, 2008), 121.

[34] Arnold, 'Vagrant India', 125.

poverty and nakedness were universal in India this did not signify the same degree of suffering as in Europe'.[35] He cites as evidence the statement of William Tennant, who was a Calcutta Chaplain: 'An Hindoo, feels himself comfortable on the same fare on which the Englishmen would languish and starve.'[36]

The 1858 Act became the legal source for the establishment and management of the lunatic asylums in India. The Magistrate, the police, and the Medical Officer played imperative roles in certifying and committing the 'native' insane to the asylum. The Act stated that 'it was the duty of the Darogah or District Police officer to send to the magistrate all persons found wandering at large within his district who were deemed to be lunatics, and all persons believed to be dangerous by the reason of lunacy'.[37] The police was to interpret alleged 'lunacy' according to the given situation. The Act indirectly made a distinction between psychiatry for the rich and for the poor. The Superintendent in Charge at the Cuttack Asylum wrote, 'Lunatics are found by the police disturbing the peace; and unable to take care of themselves, they are at once taken up and brought before the nearest magistrate.'[38] The 'wandering' and 'dangerous' lunatics were first sent to a Magistrate, who performed his medical-executive role with the help of the civil surgeon. He identified and certified insanity. After examination, the Magistrate issued orders of dispatch to the nearest jail or asylum.

Another significant aspect of the Indian Lunacy Act of 1858 was the way in which the term 'lunatic' was used. The word 'lunatic' as used in this Act 'meant and included every person of unsound mind and incapable of managing his affairs, and every person being an idiot'.[39] The definition of 'lunacy' remained vague in this period. It was left to the police and the officials to (mis)construe its meanings. Ernst aptly remarks that 'the Acts of 1858 contained material that had in England been considered as most controversial. Despite this, the discussions

---

[35] Arnold, 'Vagrant India', 121.

[36] Arnold, 'Vagrant India', 121.

[37] The Lunatic Asylums Act No. XXXVI of 1858, Clause V, NAI.

[38] Sir James Clark's Enquiry as to the Care and the Treatment of Lunatics, Home Dept./Public Branch, File No. 22–23, 19 December 1868, NAI.

[39] The Lunatic Asylums Act No. XXXVI of 1858, Clause IV, NAI.

preceding the passing of the Indian Acts were short and uncontroversial.[40] In England organizations such as the Alleged Lunatics' Friend Society and other concerned groups campaigned to limit the scope for false certification and imprisonment.[41] In India no such group existed. The Act was considered humanitarian by the colonizers, who believed that they were bringing 'science' and 'civilization' to India. Civil society in India was incipient at this stage and had other important issues to deal with. The Act of 1858 did not concern the public at large. Kolsky has rightly argued that codification in India was easy because colonial lawmakers did not face the conditions that grounded legal reform at home, such as a growing civil society and realm of public opinion.[42]

Reform and Reorganization

The IHDC in 1894 aimed to ascertain the extent of hemp cultivation, the procedures by which the hemp plant was made into a drug, the classes that were prone to the use of such a drug, and the forms of its consumption. One of the primary objectives of the commission was to investigate hemp's links to insanity since asylum statistics had time and again reiterated connections between the two.[43] Hemp was a common recreational drug used by Indians. James H. Mills argued,

> In the first half of the nineteenth century, British observers were vaguely aware of hemp as a substance that Indians used but by the end of nineteenth century the drug was increasingly viewed both as a cause and symptom of insanity. By the nineteenth century cannabis was being linked in India to sexual immorality, chronic indolence, violence and disorderly behavior.[44]

---

[40]   Ernst, *Mad Tales from the Raj*, 46.

[41]   Joseph Melling and Bill Forsythe, *The Politics of Madness: The State, Insanity and Society in England, 1845–1914* (London: Routledge, 2006), 14.

[42]   Kolsky, 'Codification and the Rule of Colonial Difference', 634.

[43]   Report of the Indian Hemp Drugs Commission 1893–1894, vol. I (Simla: Government Central Printing Office, 1894), 7.

[44]   Mills, *Madness, Cannabis and Colonialism*, 43.

It was with the IHDC that hemp and its relationship with insanity came under close scrutiny. The commissioners studied data of the asylums and in this process collected information by examining histories of the patients. They drew attention to the haphazard ways in which the inmates were categorized and the causes attributed for their alleged insanity. The Magistrate, police, and the medical personnel were under tremendous pressure to fill up the medical certificates. Ganja[45] as a cause was internalized by the staff to the extent that at times the cause 'unknown' was changed and 'ganja' as a cause was put in its place.[46] Faulty processes were unmasked at several levels. In spite of the wide-scale enquiry, the IHDC concluded that 'there was no trustworthy basis for a satisfactory and reasonably accurate opinion on the connection between hemp drugs and insanity in the asylum statistics appended to the annual report'.[47] It was argued that hemp was a part of Indian social customs and cultural traditions. Amar Farooqui asserts that the report of the Royal Commission on Opium reinforced the idea that opium if taken in moderation was not harmful and, when administered regularly in small doses, 'was actually beneficial'.[48] It would be difficult to estimate the extent to which the conclusions of the IHDC reinforced the use of hemp but the colonial state wanted uninterrupted flow of revenue from hemp cultivation and, therefore, denied any possibility of a relationship between the drug and insanity.[49]

The use of hemp for addiction was bizarre in English eyes, as in England hemp was never used for recreational purposes. Scholars who have researched the relationship between drugs and colonialism asserted

[45] The terms 'ganja', 'hemp', 'cannabis', and 'opium' have been used interchangeably in the reports cited in this chapter.

[46] Report of the Indian Hemp Drugs Commission 1893–1894, vol. I, 232.

[47] Report of the Indian Hemp Drugs Commission 1893–1894, vol. I, 237.

[48] Amar Farooqui, 'Opium as a Household Remedy in Nineteenth-Century Western India?', in *The Social History of Health and Medicine in Colonial India*, edited by Biswamoy Pati and Mark Harrison (London: Routledge, 2009), 230.

[49] Marijuana continues to be a controlled substance. It is regarded as a controversial drug as far as psychiatric disorders are concerned.

that 'drugs remained at the heart of empire'.[50] Mills and Barton, for example, regard that 'the need to find products to sell to Africans and Asians in exchange of prized commodities such as slaves and tea led Europeans to become merchants of drugs and drink, and their success in this role saw societies across the world become markets of intoxicants that have endured to this day and which changed the habits and tastes forever'.[51] Imperialism 'by encouraging this trade of drugs undermined their "civilizing" nature consequently giving way to liberals and missionaries who projected drugs users as victims that were in the need of salvation'.[52] The colonial drug policy first established links between hemp and insanity but later denied any such associations. A critical assessment of the hemp drug policy permits us to understand this urgent need to initiate asylum reforms. The asylums system was much easier to modify than the hemp drug policy and the asylum reform was possible without creating any massive financial deficit.

The colonial state directed its attention and energies towards the restructuring of the asylums system. The critique offered by the IHDC became the basis for a separate report, wherein two IHDC Commissioners, A. H. L. Fraser (Commissioner, Chhattisgarh division), and C. J. H. Warden (Professor of Chemistry, Calcutta), reflected upon the limitations of the asylum system in India. They criticized the management and organization of asylums and demanded professionalization of psychiatry. For the Commissioners, asylum work was a professional matter and in India the systematic treatment of the insane was non-existent. Having some knowledge about asylum management in England, they considered asylums in India as disordered. They revealed the miserable state of affairs by illustrating instances of maladministration and also pointed out that 'the superintendents held asylum work as an additional charge since they had other duties to perform'.[53] The asylum work fell in the hands of untrained subordinates. The Commissioners believed

[50] James H. Mills and Patricia Barton, 'Introduction', in *Drugs and Empire: Essays in Modern Imperialism and Intoxication, c. 1500–1930*, edited by James H. Mills and Patricia Barton (New York: Palgrave Macmillan, 2007), 1.

[51] Mills and Barton, 'Introduction', 1–2.

[52] Mills and Barton, 'Introduction', 1–2.

[53] Proposed Improvement in the Administration of Lunatic Asylum in India, Home Dept./Medical Branch, File No. 97–99, March 1895, NAI, 34.

that the Superintendents of asylums lacked special experience and skill in the treatment of mental diseases and were often largely disinterested.[54] It was recommended that 'whole-time superintendents should be appointed because under the prevalent system, the civil-surgeons did not have sufficient time for asylum work'.[55]

Andrew Scull argues that the reification of the professional identity of psychiatrists in England was a complex process. By 1845 the medical profession had secured powerful support for the proposition that insanity was a disease, and thus naturally something which doctors alone were qualified to treat.[56] By the mid-nineteenth century, professional psychiatric organizations had come up to secure a separate identity for the profession. The earliest of these was the Association of Medical Officers of Asylums and Hospitals for the Insane. In 1853 the Association launched its own periodical, *The Asylum Journal*. The professionalization of psychiatry was further catalysed by skill and specialty. The second half of the nineteenth century witnessed several waves of legislation related to insanity in England. The Lunacy Act of 1845 made it compulsory for every county and borough to have its own lunatic asylum for interning the mad, and a Lunacy Commission was set up in order to inspect the workings of asylums all over the country. The 1853 Act furthered the provisions of the 1845 Act. Also significant was the Act of 1890, which was enacted to prevent wrongful certification and confinement. These Acts led to the concretization of psychiatry as a discipline. Psychiatrists or 'mad-doctors' were now seen as those people who knew how to manage, identify, and certify insanity, on account of their medico-legal training. The key to understanding and curing madness was its proper management.

Jan Goldstein in her classic work *Console and Classify* looks into the making of French psychiatry as a profession in the nineteenth century. She points out:

> Among the many 'human sciences' thrown up by this far-reaching development was psychiatry, the medical study and treatment of disorders of

---

[54] Proposed Improvement in the Administration of Lunatic Asylum in India, Home Dept./Medical Branch, File No. 97–99, March 1895, NAI, 35.

[55] Proposed Improvement in the Administration of Lunatic Asylum in India, Home Dept./Medical Branch, File No. 97–99, March 1895, NAI, 35.

[56] Scull, *The Most Solitary Afflictions*, 232.

the mind. It arose almost simultaneously in France, Britain, America and the German Lands and despite considerable mutual borrowing, soon bore in each setting the mark of a distinctive national tradition. From the closing decade of the eighteenth century, when they pledged to outdistance their English rivals, to the closing decade of the nineteenth century, when they began to be overtaken by the Germans, French physicians played the singular most vigorous role in constituting and legitimising a psychiatric science.[57]

In India, this process of legitimizing and professionalizing psychiatry was slow and uneven. The insane asylums were first built during the beginning of the nineteenth century for incarcerating European soldiers but were later on extended to the 'natives'. Rules and regulations regarding the working of the asylums were formulated during the early half of the nineteenth century. These loosely defined principles that were tailored for the functioning of the asylums during the beginning of the nineteenth century became outdated by the beginning of the twentieth century since the asylums grew in number and size.

England had mammoth asylums by contrast, and there existed in India small asylums covering different regions. An important suggestion made by the IHDC commissioners was the amalgamation of small asylums in order to create bigger ones. Judging against the English asylums, they felt that the asylum staff had no skills and was not provided with any special training. The commissioners argued that the lack of training was a predicament produced due to lack of scientific study of insanity in India. Training in medical schools consisted of a few lectures on medical jurisprudence. These lectures were generally delivered by men who had 'no special experience of insanity'.[58] The Superintendent, the 'native' doctor, and the subordinate staff needed training and specialization in the mental illnesses though none of this was available. Debjani Das though points out that 'in case the individual was departing to join as a physician in one of the asylums in India, then additional training from Bethlem, St. Luke Hospital, or other hospital of a similar measure in England was

---

[57] Jan Goldstein, *Console and Classify: The French Psychiatric Profession in the Nineteenth Century* (Chicago: The University of Chicago Press, 2001), 1.

[58] Proposed Improvement in the Administration of Lunatic Asylum in India, Home Dept./Medical Branch, File No. 97–99, March 1895, NAI, 1.

considered all the more necessary'.[59] The training helped them to understand the disease but there is little evidence to support that all underwent the prescribed training. While certain Superintendents in Charge were keen to know about the disease and kept themselves updated with the new developments at home and abroad, others performed theirs duties as keepers.[60]

The Commissioners, Fraser and Warden, urged the state to initiate a proper study of insanity in India. They felt that the government was wasting resources on the small asylums and argued that asylums should be centralized in order to secure maximum efficiency while minimizing costs.[61] They believed that centralization of asylums would lead to special training in the mental diseases, as central asylums would become training grounds for subordinate staff. Reform was possible only if the government devoted special attention to the study of mental diseases in India. These solutions offered by the IHDC Commissioners were not welcomed by the government as reform and reorganization would require expenditure. A full-length report was prepared by Dr Rice (Surgeon General) offering resolutions to the problems. There was a lengthy discussion on the English precedents, first in the report of Warden and Fraser, and then in Rice's suggestions. From the very beginning, however, it was made clear that it was impossible for the colonial state to have the same psychiatric infrastructure as what existed in England. Rice remarked:

> If these are contrasted with the expensive, specially designed lunatic asylums in European countries, and specially trained whole time medical officers, sumptuously paid and housed on the premises, with assistants quite as well trained but of only less standing and experience ... with the already fully occupied Civil Surgeons [in Indian lunatic asylums] who have no previous training at all, and who have to do all the professional

---

[59] Debjani Das, *Houses of Madness: Insanity and Asylums of Bengal in Nineteenth-Century India* (New Delhi: Oxford University Press, 2015), 15.

[60] For details, see Shilpi Rajpal, 'Colonial Psychiatry in Mid-Nineteenth Century: The James Clark Enquiry', *South Asia Research*, vol. 35, no. 1 (February 2015).

[61] Proposed Improvement in the Administration of Lunatic Asylum in India, Home Dept./Medical Branch, File No. 97–99, March 1895, NAI, 35.

work themselves, I shall be surprised if it is not admitted that it cannot in reason be expected that an insane asylum can be run on the same lines in the country as at home.[62]

Historians of medicine have spoken about the limited nature of colonial medicine.[63] Rice attempted to defend the constraints of the existing establishment. He recommended reorganizing the 'native' asylums into various classes and suggested that the first-class asylums should hold 700 to 1,000 inmates, and have a whole-time Superintendent, and be established in Bombay, Bengal, and the North-Western Provinces. The second-class asylums would hold 400 to 700 inmates, and were to be established in Madras and Punjab. The latter would have a Civil Surgeon as the Superintendent.[64] He also suggested the amalgamation of existing small asylums with these first- and the second-class asylums. Another significant recommendation was that rigorous screening of lunatics be undertaken at the time of admission. This was to prevent the admission into asylums of persons suffering from the temporary result of sickness, intemperance, or debauchery, and those whom their friends ought to support.[65]

The government renounced the plan of centralizing all the asylums as local governments objected to the measure. Several small asylums were nevertheless shut down. The Delhi Asylum was permanently closed in 1899 as a new asylum was established at Lahore early in 1900 and all the patients of the Delhi Asylum—103 male patients and 35 female patients—were transferred to it.[66] Thereafter, Punjab had only a central

[62] Proposed Improvement in the Administration of Lunatic Asylum in India, Home Dept./Medical Branch, File Nos 97–9, March 1895, NAI, 1.

[63] Mark Harrison and Biswamoy Pati, 'Social History of Health and Medicine: Colonial India', in *The Social History of Health and Medicine in Colonial India*, edited by Biswamoy Pati and Mark Harrison (London: Routledge, 2009), 6.

[64] Administration of Lunatic Asylums in India, Home Dept./Medical Branch, File No. 188–232, August 1897, NAI, 1–2.

[65] Administration of Lunatic Asylums in India, Home Dept./Medical Branch, File No. 188–232, August 1897, NAI, 1–2.

[66] The Annual Report of the Lunatic Asylum of the Punjab for the Year 1900, National Medical Library, New Delhi. It should be kept in mind that Delhi was administratively part of Punjab after 1857.

lunatic asylum at Lahore. In Bengal, the Cuttack asylum was closed but the asylum in Tezpur continued to function due to the objections of the local government. In the North-Western Provinces, the Lucknow asylum was merged with the Agra asylum. The Agra asylum was declared the central asylum for the purpose of training. Although centralization was meant to initiate a process of specialization, this goal was never fully achieved. Despite chidings of members of the IHDC, the recommendations of the study of insanity was not introduced in a full-fledged manner. The central government sought views of the provincial governments about the introduction of psychiatry in the medical curriculum. The Chief Commissioner of Burma stated that 'there are many subjects of far more practical use than the study of insanity'.[67] The Bengal government argued that 'it would not be worthwhile to add a new subject to the course for the sake of training one man'.[68] Shruti Kapila has also pointed out that 'while specialization was desirable and vital for the reform of colonial psychiatry, its realisation was at odds with the general objectives of the Indian Medical Service'.[69]

In areas where there were several asylums, one asylum was selected for the purpose of lecturing. The full-time officers were specially appointed as Superintendents for these newly amalgamated asylums. Attempts were made to appoint as Superintendents those who had gained some knowledge of mental diseases in the United Kingdom. The full-time Superintendent in Charge was given an additional payment for lecturing in the medical schools. The Lahore asylum was the first to be centralized and developed as a 'modern' asylum. J. T. W. Leslie, the Director General of Medicine, wrote in an unofficial memorandum:

> In India up to now the asylums have been built on prison lines, and though the underground dungeons at Bhowanipore have not been used for many years ... I have today visited the old, and the site for the new, asylum at

[67] Administration of Lunatic Asylums in India, Home Dept./Medical Branch, File No. 188–232, August 1897, NAI, 1–2.

[68] Administration of Lunatic Asylums in India, Home Dept./Medical Branch, File No. 188–232, August 1897, NAI, 1–2.

[69] Shruti Kapila, 'The Making of Colonial Psychiatry, Bombay Presidency, 1849–1940', unpublished doctoral thesis, School of Oriental and African Studies, University of London, 2002, 96.

Lahore. The old one is a *serai* adapted for the purposes of the safe keeping of lunatics on strict prison lines ... The new asylum, though it will be a great improvement on the old one, is planned on the same lines *and will be nothing more than a somewhat glorified prison* (emphasis added).[70]

He advocated the development of psychiatry along the lines of modern European asylums. He felt that restraint should be dispensed with and that all walls and bars should be abolished.

The turn of the twentieth century witnessed changes but in many ways old methods and practices continued. The so-called reforms and reorganization had inherent limitations for which reasons these became ineffective in a decade or two. The obsolete patterns were quite visible in the ways reform was structured. In fact, it would not be wrong to argue that reform was a manoeuvre on the part of the government to direct the attention from hemp to asylums. It was an intelligently devised mechanism to ensure the incessant flow of revenue. The reform and amalgamation of asylums were in fact seen as a cost-saving measure. The mammoth asylums soon became unmanageable in the absence of modern facilities and trained staff. C. J. Lodge Patch, the Superintendent in Charge of the Lahore asylum, described his first visit to that asylum in 1922 in the following words:

> Nearly all the male patients were allowed to go about stark naked without even a loincloth; handcuffs and fetters are applied on the slightest provo-cation or without apparent provocation by any attendant who cared to use mechanical restraint, and universal seclusion was the part of the daily routine ... my first action was to collect two hundredweight of handcuffs and other instruments of torture and send them in a bullock-cart to the Central jail.[71]

The government wished to devise reforms that were financially viable. Every attempt made to reform and reorganize had the latent intent of economizing. Similar attempts of economizing also took place in England during the same period. Scull argues that 'the practice of cheeseparing

[70] Plans for the New Central Asylum to be constructed at Lahore, Home/Medical, November 1898, File No. 139–140, NAI.

[71] C. J. Lodge Patch, 'A Century of Psychiatry in the Punjab', *Journal of Mental Science*, vol. 70 (1930): 389.

worked through overcrowding of pauper lunatics and increase in intake of paying patients.[72] Nonetheless, the process of closing down of the small asylums and opening of centralized ones was peculiar to India. Economizing through centralization impeded all possibility of further developments. Mammoth asylums were common in Europe but facilities that enabled their management there were entirely absent in India. It can be argued that modernization along the lines of English psychiatry was only a cover-up that the colonial state used occasionally as a rhetoric to demonstrate liberality and advancement.

Anouska Bhattachayya locates 'the emergence of the specialised knowledge in macro-administrative change, attempts to converge or delineate medical and judicial spheres and publication of the new genre of the lunacy text'.[73] She fails to situate the significant role the reform cycle played during the turn of century. Shruti Kapila emphasizes the interesting links between the IHDC and asylum reorganization. She argues that 'questions of "reform" of the working of the colonial psychiatry, at the beginning of the twentieth century were in the language of "professionalism", "specialism", and "scientific" culture. The agenda of government more than fifty years on, in relation to the disciplinary agendas of psychiatry was then, to recast them along the "improved lines of modern practice"'.[74] Kapila aptly points out that the 'questions of economy overrode any considerations of efficacy of the reform and professionalisation of the institutional identity of colonial psychiatry'.[75] In other words, the reform cycle that was initiated during the beginning of the twentieth century was devised to maintain financial stringency. Samiksha Sehrawat sheds light on the need of budgeting the medical expenditure in case of hospitals. She points out,

> Private philanthropic effort was considered the proper motor for the construction and maintenance of voluntary hospitals in nineteenth century Britain ... the colonial state's initiative to found dispensaries in India did

[72] Scull, *The Most Solitary Afflictions*.

[73] Anouska Bhattacharyya, 'Indian Insanes: Lunacy in the "Native" Asylums of Colonial India, 1858–1912', unpublished doctoral thesis, Harvard University, 2013, 175.

[74] Kapila, 'The Making of Colonial Psychiatry', 82.

[75] Kapila, 'The Making of Colonial Psychiatry', 88.

not indicate the abandoning of these principles but rather the launching of an improving project for Indian society. Thus, the colonial state's participation in medical philanthropy was meant to 'stimulate' its colonial subject to emulation of British ideals of voluntary associational culture and utilitarian philosophy.[76]

The asylum system during the nineteenth century was an integral part of the punitive order. Philanthropy on the large scale was not much of an option since asylums throughout the nineteenth century were peopled by the poor, since the rich and the middle classes looked down upon these incarceral institutions. The state initiative to reform had the latent intent of privatizing psychiatric care over the period. According to the 1912 Act, the reception of a petition had to be submitted by the husband or wife or the nearest relative of the patient,[77] since it was believed that this would prevent the illegal detention of the sane. The new requirements made it impossible for the poor to admit their relatives as submitting the application was a costly and time-consuming process. The only way the poor could avail of the facility was by leaving their relatives on the streets. The poor who were regarded as 'troubled' could be picked up by the police whereas the rich had to submit an application and pay for their stay. The division between the psychiatry for the rich and the poor was, therefore, complete.

'Lunatic' Asylums or 'Mental' Hospitals

The twentieth century was a period of flux in the history of psychiatry in India. The state made attempts to revamp the psychiatric infrastructure in the period. The 1912 Act was a significant attempt to consolidate lunacy laws. This period also witnessed changes due to individual efforts. These individuals were usually (though not always) Superintendents in charge of the central asylums. Individuals for the first time loomed large on the scene of the history of psychiatry of India. The IHDC's condemnation of the asylum system in India had led to the centralization of the institutions in Calcutta, Poona, Madras, Agra, Lahore, and

---

[76] Samiksha Sehrawat, *Colonial Medical Care in North India: Gender, State, and Society, c. 1840–1920* (Delhi: Oxford University Press, 2013), 14–15.

[77] Chapter II, Section 6, The Indian Lunacy Act No. IV of 1912, NAI.

Rangoon. These institutions had full-time Superintendents who were capable of managing such central asylums. The notion that the central asylums would become centres for the study of insanity paved the way for their specialization. The scientific study of insanity never took off on a larger scale. Nonetheless, the concept of a specialist emerged during this period. Some of these specialists dedicated their lives to the cause of studying insanity and some of the central asylums became hubs for psychiatric deliberations. These deliberations were often among the individuals and the colonial state. These negotiations were sometimes successful but failed at other times. What should be kept in mind is that innovation and interest depended entirely on the zeal of the Superintendent in Charge. His motivation was his own as the government did not have much stake in the process. The change also included bringing psychiatry in India in line with international developments in the field. These changes, however, should not be understood in terms of teleological growth.

The changes that were triggered due to IHDC criticism began making a visible difference in altering the psychiatric infrastructure. Kapila also points out that 'criticism and rhetoric of reform nevertheless resulted in the recognition of the realm of colonial psychiatry distinct from both penology and other medical disciplines'.[78] During this period the question of alteration in nomenclature from 'lunatic asylum' to 'mental hospital' was interlinked with the question of curative treatment. Curative treatment was scarce in the lunatic asylums. Asylum as a term meant a place that was a 'refuge' or 'safe haven' for lunatics. These 'safe havens' were built to keep the public safe from the 'dangerous' insane. According to Michel Foucault '"Dangerousness" meant that the individual "must be considered at the level of his potentialities (*ses virtualites*) and not the level of his acts," not as someone who had actually violated the law, but as someone whose potential behaviour had to be subject to subject to control and correction'.[79] By the end of the century, pessimism related to the cure rates of insanity had heightened. The asylums in the West were filled with 'incurables' as the number of 'cured' patients had

[78] Kapila, 'The Making of Colonial Psychiatry', 98.
[79] Michel Foucault, *Abnormal: Lectures at the College de France 1974–75*, translated by by Graham Burchell (New Delhi: Navayana, 2010), xxiii.

dropped. Moral therapy came to be regarded as redundant as psychiatry took a biological turn.

By the end of the century, the term 'lunatic' was considered offensive and the word 'asylum' had also become outmoded. In England, the term 'lunatic asylum' was replaced with the word 'mental hospital'. The change in the terminology should be understood in terms of the shift in the knowledge systems regarding the disease and its cure. The Government of India was neither interested in any further reorganization of psychiatry nor in the change of nomenclature. This is evidenced by the fact that the Government of India took more than ten years to resolve the issue of whether the nomenclature 'lunatic asylum' ought to be changed to 'mental hospital' or not. Discussions regarding the change of the terminology reveal covert attitudes of the state and bureaucracy. P. Hefferman, the Superintendent of the Madras Lunatic Asylum, was the first one to suggest that 'the term "lunatic" is a relic of a barbarous age'.[80] He further pointed out:

> A gentleman who was treated in this institution in the present year, and made a good recovery, a clergy man wrote to me a short time ago and suggested that I should petition government to change the name of the institution to that of the 'MADRAS MENTAL INFIRMARY'. I cordially agreed with him and seize the present occasion to carry his suggestion into effect.[81]

In 1917 the governments of Madras, Bengal, Punjab, Burma, the Central Provinces, Assam, and Coorg accepted the proposal to change the designation 'lunatic asylum' to 'mental hospital'. The proposal was opposed by the Government of United Provinces. S. P. O. Donnell, the Secretary to Government of the United Provinces, wrote to the Secretary to the Government of India:

> The term 'lunatic asylum' is a much more accurate description of the institution referred to than 'Mental Hospital' would be. Curative

---

[80] From Captain P. Hefferman, Superintendent, Madras Lunatic Asylum to the Personal Assistant to the Surgeon General with the Government of Madras, the papers related to the Indian Lunacy Acts No. IV of 1912, NAI.

[81] From Captain P. Hefferman, Superintendent, Madras Lunatic Asylum to the Personal Assistant to the Surgeon General with the Government of Madras, the papers related to the Indian Lunacy Acts No. IV of 1912, NAI.

treatment is not at present the primary object of the existence of the asylum in the United Provinces. The aim and the purpose of these institutions is rather to provide accommodation where lunatics are dangerous to themselves or to others who are a nuisance to the community and can be kept in safe custody under reasonable, comfortable and healthy conditions; it would be impossible to convert them into hospitals designed primarily for the treatment without the introduction of changes which would be extremely costly ... the change of designation would be misleading.[82]

The perspective of Donnell reflects the nature of colonial psychiatry. The aim was largely to incarcerate the mad and the delinquent whereas 'cure' as a notion was sidelined in general. W. M. Hailey, the Chief Commissioner of Delhi, argued that 'whatever name we give to the institution it will still be the "*Pagal Khana*" for Indians, and disinclination to commit a friend or relative to its care will not be affected by a change in its official designation'.[83] Sarah Ann Pinto has argued that 'the elite eluded the asylum because it lacked scientific methods of treatment ... the middle class and the poor also avoided the use of the asylum' because of the process of admission and incarceration. Most patients in the asylums were 'found committing mischief in the public streets and [were] caught and conveyed [to the asylum] by the police'.[84]

The Indian Lunacy Act of 1912 was amended in 1922, and this amendment allowed for the much desired change in the designation of 'lunatic asylum' to 'mental hospital'. The bill for the Act stated that 'it is, however, necessary to retain the word "asylum" in the Act, because of its

[82] From S. P. O. Donnell, the Secretary to the Government of the United Province, to the Secretary to the Government of India Proposal that the Designation 'Lunatic Asylum' Should Be Changed to 'Mental Hospital', Home/Medical, File No. 96–106, May 1917, NAI.

[83] From W. M. Hailey, the Chief Commissioner of Delhi, to the Secretary to the Government of India, Home Department, Proposal that the Designation 'Lunatic Asylum' Should Be Changed to 'Mental Hospital', Home/Medical, File No. 96–106, May 1917, NAI.

[84] Sarah Ann Pinto, 'Shackled Bodies Unchained Minds: Lunatic Asylums in the Bombay Presidency, 1793–1921', unpublished doctoral thesis, Victoria University of Wellington, 2017, 6.

use in other legislation'.[85] After much debate the 'lunatic asylums' were designated as 'mental hospitals'. This change in nomenclature called for reform at least in theory, if not practice. In a discussion over the passing of the bill, the following was stated:

> It has also been pointed out though medical treatment is actually given in some asylums still the present designation deters people from availing themselves to it. The government of India appreciate the purpose of the proposed change in designation and they recognise the importance of emphasising the curative treatment which should be available in these institutions.[86]

The government of India was aware of the situation as it stated clearly that 'medical treatment is actually given in *some* [emphasis added] asylums'.[87] Act IV of 1922 added to section 84 of the 1912 Lunacy Act the following qualification: 'if it is satisfied that provision has been or will be made for the curative treatment therein of persons suffering from mental diseases'.[88] The amendment stated that 'if in any licensed asylum no provision for curative treatment has been made, or the Local Government may consider that the provision made is insufficient, the Local Government may require the person in charge of the asylum to take such measures for making or supplementing such provision'.[89] No licensed asylums existed in this period. Curative treatment at least officially had become the norm.

Some serious efforts were made to organize the psychiatric services in the period by these emerging specialists. The waves of change were

[85] The Statement of Objects and Reasons, The Indian Lunacy (Amendment) Act, 1922 (Act IV of 1922), Legislative/Assembly and Council Branch, File No. 52–60, June 1922, NAI.

[86] The Indian Lunacy (Amendment) Act, 1922 (Act IV of 1922), Legislative/Assembly and Council Branch, File No. 52–60, June 1922, NAI.

[87] The Indian Lunacy (Amendment) Act, 1922 (Act IV of 1922), Legislative/Assembly and Council Branch, File No. 52–60, June 1922, NAI.

[88] The Indian Lunacy (Amendment) Act, 1922 (Act IV of 1922), Legislative/Assembly and Council Branch, File No. 52–60, June 1922, NAI.

[89] The Indian Lunacy (Amendment) Act, 1922 (Act IV of 1922), Legislative/Assembly and Council Branch, File No. 52–60, June 1922, NAI.

experienced, articulated, and demanded by a small group of individuals. The term 'professionalization' has been described by Thomas Broman as a set of criteria that usually included '(1) specialized and advanced education; (2) a code of conduct or ethics; (3) competency tests leading to licensing; (4) high social prestige in comparison to manual labour; (5) monopolization of the market in services; and (6) considerable autonomy in conduct of professional affairs'.[90] The want of a professional body and specialized training was articulated by psychiatrists. England had a professional body called the Board of Commissioners from the mid-nineteenth century. In India this need for the professional body and special education to train psychiatrists was expressed by W. S. J. Shaw, the Superintendent of the Yeravda Central Asylum, Pune. He clamoured for the need to reorganize lunacy administration in India. For a whole decade Shaw made several appeals to the Government of India that the Alienist[91] Department was essential for the proper functioning of asylums. He remarked that 'the government has been considering the formation of an organized department since 1906 but nothing was been done so far'.[92] He noted that such an organized department would include all the grades of asylum officials: Superintendents, Assistant Medical Officers (in various grades), nurses, attendants, stewards, clerks, and such others. He was convinced that no advancement in the administration of psychiatry in India was likely to occur until an organized 'Department of Psychiatry' was established. Individual psychiatrists, such as Shaw, had self-interests at stake but were also interested in the greater change.

Shaw contended that 'the cost of organizing the department would be modest and an organized department would amend the overall

[90] Thomas Broman, 'Rethinking Professionalization: Theory, Practice, and Professional Ideology in Eighteenth-Century German Medicine', *The Journal of Modern History*, vol. 67, no. 4 (1995): 835.

[91] Andrew Scull has described that the English term 'mad-doctor' was replaced by the French word *alieniste*. The word 'alienist' was changed by the German term 'psychiatrist'. For details, see Andrew Scull, *Hysteria: The Disturbing History* (Oxford: Oxford University Press, 2009), 191.

[92] Proposals for Improving the Administration of Lunatic Asylums and for Constitution of a Separate Alienist Department in India, Home/Jail, File No 144, 1923, NAI.

administration of lunacy in India.[93] Berkeley-Hill, the Superintendent of the Ranchi European Lunatic Asylum, concurred with Shaw's proposal regarding the formation of an organized Alienist Department. He wrote to the Inspector General of Civil Hospitals, Bihar and Orissa, that the 'time has arrived for the introduction of radical changes in the organisation, equipment and administration of lunatic asylums in India.'[94] Berkeley-Hill felt that 'the most urgent motive, in India as well as elsewhere, for the institutions of this type is to serve as teaching centres for psychiatric training.'[95] He appealed for the establishment of specialized hospitals for observation, treatment, research, and training. Berkeley-Hill suggested that the men of the same class as those who were lecturers on mental diseases in the medical schools in England and America should be recruited. These alienists were expected to train Indians with superior medical qualifications locally for work in the alienist department.[96] He also added to the debate on the insane that the central asylums should be styled as mental hospitals as 'the word asylum frightens them [the people] and keeps them away' and that there was serious stigma attached to this term.[97]

[93] From W. S. J. Shaw, Superintendent, Central Asylum, Yeravda, to the Personal Assistant to the Surgeon General with the Government of Bombay, Poona, Proposals for Improving the Administration of Lunatic Asylums and for Constitution of a Separate Alienist Department in India, Home/Jails, File No 144, 1923, NAI.

[94] From Berkeley-Hill, Superintendent, Ranchi European Mental Hospital to the Inspector General of Civil Hospitals, Bihar and Orissa, Proposals for Improving the Administration of Lunatic Asylums and for Constitution of a Separate Alienist Department in India, Home/Jails, File No 144, 1923, NAI.

[95] From Berkeley-Hill, Superintendent, Ranchi European Mental Hospital to the Inspector General of Civil Hospitals, Bihar and Orissa, Proposals for Improving the Administration of Lunatic Asylums and for Constitution of a Separate Alienist Department in India, Home/Jails, File No 144, 1923, NAI.

[96] From Berkeley-Hill, Superintendent, Ranchi European Mental Hospital to the Inspector General of Civil Hospitals, Bihar and Orissa, Proposals for Improving the Administration of Lunatic Asylums and for Constitution of a Separate Alienist Department in India, Home/Jails, File No 144, 1923, NAI.

[97] From Berkeley-Hill, Superintendent, Ranchi European Mental Hospital to the Inspector General of Civil Hospitals, Bihar and Orissa, Proposals for Improving the Administration of Lunatic Asylums and for Constitution of a Separate Alienist Department in India, Home/Jails, File No 144, 1923, NAI.

Shaw had similar concerns and he mentioned that 'there is at present practically no proper system of education in psychiatry'.[98] He wrote the 'Memorandum on Lunacy Administration in India',[99] in which he commented that 'there is no committee or central body in India similar to the Board of Commissioners in England to supervise the administration of the Indian lunacy Act'.[100] He reiterated the urgent need for trained staff and the difficulties faced in securing specialists, and urged the Government to create a department for alienists. His appeals regarding the creation of a specialist department were rejected. It was stated that 'this cannot be done, and no further action seems to be necessary'.[101] Shaw raised the matter again after a gap of two years. He recalled that at the time of his appointment 'in 1906 the alienist department was supposed to have been initiated by the instance of the Secretary of State, and medical officers interested in psychiatry were attracted to the department as the "*pucca*" one'.[102] He remarked 'as I have represented, no real effort has since been made to carry out the idea, and now it is admitted that the "Department" does not exist'.[103] He urged 'in

[98] From W. S. J. Shaw, Superintendent, Central Asylum, Yeravda, to the Personal Assistant to the Surgeon General with the Government of Bombay, Poona, Proposals for Improving the Administration of Lunatic Asylums and for Constitution of a Separate Alienist Department in India, Home/Jail, File No. 144, 1923, NAI.

[99] Memorandum on Lunacy Administration in India by W. S. J. Shaw, Superintendent of the Central Mental Hospital at Yeravda, Bombay Presidency, Home/Jail, File No. 103/24, 1924, NAI.

[100] Memorandum on Lunacy Administration in India by W. S. J. Shaw, Superintendent of the Central Mental Hospital at Yeravda, Bombay Presidency, Home/Jail, File No. 103/24, 1924, NAI.

[101] Memorandum on Lunacy Administration in India by W. S. J. Shaw, Superintendent of the Central Mental Hospital at Yeravda, Bombay Presidency, Home/Jail, File No. 103/24, 1924, NAI.

[102] Memorandum on Lunacy Administration in India by W. S. J. Shaw, Superintendent of the Central Mental Hospital at Yeravda, Bombay Presidency, Home/Jail, File No. 103/24, 1924, NAI.

[103] Memorandum on Lunacy Administration in India by W. S. J. Shaw, Superintendent of the Central Mental Hospital at Yeravda, Bombay Presidency, Home/Jail, File No. 103/24, 1924, NAI.

the name of humanity and efficiency, to recommend a reconsideration of the disposal of my "memorandum".[104] Shaw requested that his suggestion be forwarded to the Secretary of State. His request was declined and it was pointed out that 'the administration of the mental hospital is a provincial matter transferred over, on which the secretary of state can exercise superintendence, direction and control only for a very limited purposes, which are here irrelevant.[105] The local governments had argued against the proposal on grounds of financial stringency. L. S. White, Deputy Secretary to the Government of the United Provinces, Judicial Department, wrote to the Secretary to the Government of India, Home Department, that 'under the present circumstances, it has been found impossible to provide the necessary funds and the proposal must inevitably be deferred till the financial condition of these is more satisfactory.[106]

By the turn of the century, the mental hospitals in England, America, and Europe had become pinnacles of innovation and new therapies emerged. However, the Government of India did not take any concrete steps to medicalize psychiatry and a host of other indigenous therapies continued to flourish alongside Western medicine. In India, mental illness was regarded as no less than a crime. The period 1905 to 1922 witnessed the rise of nationalism as a movement in India.[107]

---

[104] From W. S. J. Shaw to the Surgeon General with the Government of Bombay, Memorandum of Lieut. Col. W. S. J. Shaw, I. M. S. on the Lunacy Administration in India, Home/Jails, File No. 529, 1926, NAI.

[105] From J. E. Dunnett, the Joint Secretary to the Government of Bombay, to the Secretary to the Government of Bombay, Memorandum of Lieut. Col. W. S. J. Shaw, I. M. S. on the Lunacy Administration in India, File No. 529, Home/Jail, 1926, NAI.

[106] From L. S. White, Deputy Secretary to the Government of the United Provinces, Judicial Department, to the Secretary to the Government of India, Home Department, Proposals for Improving the Administration of Lunatic asylums and for constitution of a separate Alienist Department in India, Home/Jail, File No. 144, 1923, NAI.

[107] Also see Sumit Sarkar, *The Swadeshi Movement in Bengal 1903–1908*, new edition with a preface by the author and critical essays by Neeladri Bhattacharya and Dipesh Chakrabarty (Ranikhet: Permanent Black, 2010, first ed. 1973).

The devolution of powers to local governments was a result of this intensified struggle. The unrest began with the partition of Bengal in 1905 and the surge of the swadeshi movement. Sumit Sarkar argues that 'there was first what may be termed "constructive *swadeshi*"—the rejection of futile and self-demeaning "mendicant" politics in favor of self-help through Swadeshi industries, national schools and attempts at village improvements and organisation'.[108] The Indian Councils Act of 1909 allowed Indians to contest elections for the legislative council. It allowed greater powers for budget discussion, raising questions, and sponsoring resolutions to members of legislative councils, who were to be elected on the basis of a highly restrictive and divisive franchise for the first time. These measures were not acceptable to many sections of Indian nationalists, and were the most short-lived of all early constitutional 'reforms'. They had to be revised in ten years.[109] The devolution of power was further made possible with the Government of India Act of 1919. The Act laid the basis for 'dyarchy', which meant that certain functions were 'transferred' to the provincial governments, while others were kept 'reserved'. Health, education, and agriculture were transferred to the provincial governments.[110]

Although health was a subject that was 'transferred' to provincial governments under the 1919 Act, this did not bring changes in the overall system. The entry of Indians into the upper echelons of the administration was slow. The mere idea that Indians could be now admitted into the Indian Medical Service (IMS) made colonial officials anxious. In 1921, W. B. Brander, Secretary to the Government of Bombay, wrote to the Secretary to the Government of India:

> Services under the government of India has [have] not now those attractions which it once had. Variations of exchange, the limitations imposed by the government system, the increasing feeling that posts, even in the specialized departments, should be filled entirely by Indians, contribute to a sense of unsettlement amongst European Government

---

[108] Sumit Sarkar, *Modern India: 1885–1947* (Delhi: Macmillan India, 1983), 113.

[109] Sekhar Bandyopadhyay, *From Plassey to Partition: A History of Modern India* (New Delhi: Orient Blackswan, 2004), 281.

[110] Bandyopadhyay, *From Plassey to Partition*, 283–4.

servants and detract from those merits which services in India previously possessed.[111]

This perception can be understood in the context of the fact that Indians
were now entering government services in comparatively larger numbers.
Roger Jeffery points out that 'after the 1919 Act there were long discussions on how many IMS men the provinces had to employ, and in
which posts, and each round of discussions concluded with fewer posts
remaining closed to outside competition.'[112] There was a growing need
for trained staff that could work under the specialist European. Lunacy
administration fell under the transferred list but this did not change the
scenario. Very few Indians were allowed to fill higher posts such as that
of the Superintendent in Charge of the central lunatic asylums. Indians
were denied access to the higher posts because they supposedly lacked
the necessary training.

Ernst highlights that by the mid-twentieth century an Indian
Superintendent in Charge of the Ranchi Indian Mental Hospital was
extremely successful in running it. Jal Edulji Dhunjiboy, the said medical official, travelled widely in Europe. He familiarized himself with the
latest methods of treatment and applied them to the patients of the
hospital. Ernst noted:

> When the building work at the new institution in Ranchi was completed,
> Dhunjibhoy was appointed as its first Superintendent. An appointment
> such as that at Ranchi was highly coveted among doctors. Not only did it
> entail taking over a large, brand-new purpose-built institution, but well-
> paid vacancies at senior-management level were few and far between,
> especially at a time of financial retrenchment such as the decades follow-
> ing the First World War. What is more, Dhunjibhoy was among the first
> few 'native' medical officers to head a major medical institution.[113]

---

[111] From W. B. Brander, the Secretary to the Government of Bombay,
to the Secretary to the Government of India, Proposals for Improving the
Administration of Lunatic Asylums and for Constitution of a Separate Alienist
Department in India, 1923, Home/Jail, File No 144, 1923, NAI.

[112] Roger Jeffery, 'Recognizing India's Doctors: The Institutionalization of
Medical Dependency', Modern Asian Studies, vol. 13, no. 2 (1979): 311.

[113] Waltraud Ernst, Colonialism and Transnational Psychiatry: The Development of an Indian Mental Hospital in British India, c. 1925–1940 (London:
Anthem Press, 2013), 4.

'Indianization' was a slow process and Indians who succeeded in entering higher positions invariably faced racial discrimination. Ernst argues that structural inequalities continued to persist even in terms of salaries, allowance, and status. She remarks, 'the Indianization of the colonial service was certainly an important official step towards equality—but it was an "equality" that maintained de facto discrimination against the higher sections of Indian society by means of special allowances' and recognized the services of lower-grade Indians on the basis of their closeness to European staff.[114] Dhunjiboy was paid less and faced discrimination and derision from his European colleagues.

Indians were never given the status of citizens and were regarded as subjects of British colonial state. Indians entered into the higher echelons of the government service during the twentieth century because of the intensifying nationalist struggle. Dhunjibhoy was among the fortunate few who were given the charge of mental hospitals so early on. The rest had to wait up till the late 1930s to climb up the ladder of hierarchy because of their skin colour.

Racial discrimination not only created obstructions in the process of Indianization but also delayed the progress of specialization and professionalization of Indian psychiatrists and psychiatry. There were only a few Indian psychiatrists with such names as Sharma, Das, Vaidya, Ahmad, and Rizvi before a decade had passed after Independence. It is difficult to single out their achievements. Nonetheless, by the last decade of the twentieth century, many of them were working hand-in-hand with their European counterparts to advance the cause of psychiatry.

In 1932, Shaw wrote an article titled 'The Alienist Department of India' in the *Journal of Mental Sciences* where he critiqued the existing system of psychiatric services. He stressed that the creation of an Alienist Department had been impeded again and again and pointed out that the classification of insanity in India had become obsolete. He felt that the asylums and prisons were alike in India, and remarked, 'The architecture and fittings of asylums were as a rule gaol-like, and difficult to associate with anything of the nature of a hospital, and the "keeper" staff organisation is unsatisfactory type, being modelled on that of the

---

[114] Ernst, *Colonialism and Transnational Psychiatry*, 6.

Prison Department.'[115] He concluded, 'We must continue to depend on the influence and energy of few and scattered provincial specialists for the enlightening of the politicians in the methods of civilization, during the continued absence of the central supervision contemplated in 1906.'[116] Shaw's efforts are laudable as he made several attempts to reorganize lunacy administration in India. However, being part and parcel of the empire, he was not able to critique imperialism. He blamed Indians 'since no Indian outside the I. M. S. has materially assisted in that progress'.[117] Shaw further remarked that 'the noisy section of the population led by M. K. Gandhi prefer the ayurvedic and other indigenous systems to modern methods of treatment. These so-called "systems" are based on very primitive ideas of anatomy and physiology, and are even more out-of-date than that of Galen'.[118] He also believed that 'Europeans, and persons of European habits, should not as a rule be treated in the same mental hospitals as Indians'.[119] Shaw's views were a product of his culture and time. He once wrote that 'many Indians appear to be interested in psychology, but curiously yet I have to hear of one who has taken up the subject from its pathological aspect'.[120] This fact is understandable as psychology grew outside the control and confines of the colonial state.

Professionalization and Internationalism

International movements became significant factors that determined the course of psychiatry's development in the last three decades before India's Independence. The international health movements interconnected the metropole, the colonies, and the world. The political climate

[115] W. S. J. Shaw, 'The Alienist Department in India', *Journal of Mental Sciences*, vol. 78 (1932): 332.

[116] Shaw, 'The Alienist Department in India': 341.

[117] Shaw, 'The Alienist Department in India': 341.

[118] Shaw, 'The Alienist Department in India': 334.

[119] Shaw, 'The Alienist Department in India': 333.

[120] From W. S. J. Shaw, Superintendent, Central Asylum, Yervada, to the Personal Assistant to the Surgeon General with the Government of Bombay, Poona, Proposals for Improving the Administration of Lunatic Asylums and for Constitution of a Separate Alienist Department in India, Home/Jail, 1923, File No. 144, 1923, NAI.

had changed and the metropoles were reluctantly and slowly forced to introduce recent developments in the field of science and medicine. Volker Roelcke, Paul J. Weindling, and Louis Westwood argued that by late nineteenth and early twentieth century psychiatry had become one of 'the most contested and influential modern sciences'.[121] The international relations and transfers of concepts, practices, personnel, as well as funds in a context of rising internationalism and nationalism became significant factors in shaping psychiatric development at the local and the global levels.[122]

Berkeley-Hill published an article in the journal of *Indian Medical Gazette* in 1923 where he appealed for initiating the mental hygiene movement in India.[123] He pointed out that the year 1922 marked a watershed in the history of psychiatry since the Indian Government changed the nomenclature of 'lunatic' asylums to 'mental' hospitals. This, he declared, meant a lot to those who had demanded such a change. Berkeley-Hill, however, felt that this change would mean nothing if there was a failure in altering the larger structure. He complained that 'in many of the largest towns in this country there is not a single specially qualified physician to whom a mental case can be referred for advice and treatment'.[124] Berkeley-Hill remarked in this context that in 1916 the National Committee of Mental Hygiene had been founded in the United States of America (USA), which worked for the conservation of mental health. He felt that the committee was doing great service by disseminating knowledge regarding mental diseases. England and France had followed the lead of the USA by encouraging the mental hygiene movement in their respective countries.[125] Something of a similar nature

---

[121] Volker Roelcke et al., eds, *International Relations in Psychiatry: Britain, Germany, & The United States to World War II* (Rochester: University of Rochester Press, 2010), 1.

[122] Roelcke et al., *International Relations in* Psychiatry, 1.

[123] Owen A. R. Berkeley-Hill, 'A Plea for the Inception of a Mental Hygiene Movement in India', *Indian Medical Gazette*, vol. 58, no. 6 (1923): 242–4.

[124] Berkeley-Hill, 'A Plea for the Inception of a Mental Hygiene Movement': 242–3.

[125] Berkeley-Hill, 'A Plea for the Inception of a Mental Hygiene Movement': 243–4.

ought to be initiated in India. Psychiatric knowledge should be spread by medical students among the intelligent residents of large towns. Berkeley-Hill argued that the money spent on the pursuit of spreading awareness would help in the prevention of mental disorder and the state would then spend less on the insane and their treatment.[126]

The term 'mental hygiene' dates back to the mid-nineteenth century. In 1893 Isaac Ray, founder of the American Psychiatric Association, defined it as 'the art of preserving the mind against all incidents and influences'. Adolph Meyer and Clifford Beers were two significant advocates of the mental hygiene movement in the context of the USA.[127] Adolf Meyer was a psychiatrist who believed that besides being a medical problem, mental hygiene was a civic responsibility.[128] Beers was a patient who after his recovery wrote his autobiography titled *A Mind That Found Itself*. His autobiography brought him immediate recognition and fame and he became an exponent of the mental hygiene movement. Norman Dain in his biography of Clifford W. Beers remarks that 'the mental health movement was for Beers an extension of himself, a creative responsive to his experiences and needs'.[129] Meyers and Beers believed that processes of industrialization and urbanization were undermining the mental health of Americans.[130] Beers founded the National Committee of Mental Hygiene (NCMH) in 1908. The main objective of the NCMH was to encourage the institutional growth of the movement and to change public attitudes towards the insane, and ultimately to educate the public to enable them to lead mentally healthy lives.[131] Nick Crossley also asserted that mental disorder was believed to

[126] Berkeley-Hill, 'A Plea for the Inception of a Mental Hygiene Movement': 244.

[127] Nick Crossley, *Contesting Psychiatry: Social Movements in Mental Health* (London: Routledge, 2006), 62–3.

[128] Barbara A. Dreyer, 'Adolf Meyer and Mental Hygiene: An Ideal for Public Health', *American Journal of Public Health*, vol. 76, no. 10 (1976): 1000.

[129] Norman Dain, *Clifford W. Beers: Advocate for the Insane* (Pittsburgh: University of Pittsburgh Press, 1980), 324.

[130] Crossley, *Contesting Psychiatry*, 63.

[131] Mathew Thomas, 'Mental Hygiene as an International Movement', in *International Health Organisations and Movements1918–1939*, edited by Paul Weindling et al. (Cambridge: Cambridge University Press, 1995), 284.

be linked to moral decline, particularly amongst the working class.[132] By the 1920s the mental hygiene movement had become an international movement.[133]

Berkeley-Hill was an exponent of the mental hygiene movement in India. In 1928, he started the Indian Association of Mental Hygiene, for which the British Association of Mental Hygiene was the model.[134] India was invited to the First International Hygiene Conference which was to be held at Washington in May 1930. Since Berkeley-Hill had attended the International Conference on Psychology a year earlier, it was decided that Major J. E. Dhunjibhoy, the Superintendent of Ranchi Indian Mental Hospital, would be the delegate of the Government of India.[135] Berkeley-Hill was the first president of the Indian Association of Mental Hygiene and a significant figure in the history of modern psychiatry of India. Ashis Nandy avowed that the 'Berkeley-Hill's name is inextricably linked to ... modern psychiatry and psychoanalysis in India.'[136] The Calcutta section of the association opened a psychiatric outpatient clinic on 1 May 1933 in a general hospital. Girindrasekhar Bose played an important role in running this outpatient clinic. This may be regarded as the first outpatient clinic in India for the treatment of mental disorders.[137] Berkeley-Hill worked hard to run the association. He argued that mental hygiene ought to be integrated with general medicine and education. He believed that 'if the public know more about the danger signals of approaching mental breakdown and psychiatric assistance was not delayed in such cases, what tragedies might be

---

[132] Crossley, *Contesting Psychiatry*, 63.

[133] Thomas, 'Mental Hygiene as an International Movement', 298.

[134] Christine Hartnack, *Psychoanalysis in Colonial India* (New Delhi: Oxford University Press, 2001), 32.

[135] Question to the Legislative Assembly by Rev. J. E. Chatterjee regarding India's Representation at the First International Congress on Mental Hygiene to be Held at Washington in May 1930, Home/Jails, File No. 9/1930, 1930, NAI.

[136] Ashis Nandy, *The Savage Freud and Other Essays on Possible and Retrievable Selves* (Princeton: Princeton University Press, 1995), 96.

[137] Gauranga Banerjee, 'First Psychiatric Clinic in a General Hospital in India', *Mental Health Reviews*, 2001, available at http://www.psyplexus.com/excl/fpcg.html, accessed on 15 August 2012.

avoided!'[138] Hans Pols pointed out that 'mental hygienists considered mental health as an essential condition to meet the demands of citizenship (and mental disorder as one of the main causes of social disorder). Because mental hygienists explicitly connected the mental health of individuals to national and, later, international concerns, mental hygiene activities appeared to be relevant to broader social and political goals.'[139] The mental hygiene movement was the precursor to the mental health movement. India's participation in the mental hygiene movement is significant as it gave India an edge in this field.

The dissemination of psychology and psychoanalysis in India is one of the hallmarks of the development of psychiatry and its related disciplines. Ashis Nandy remarked that 'perhaps in no other country was psychoanalysis to register such easy dominance as in India.'[140] The Department of Psychology was established in 1915 in the University of Calcutta. Psychology initially grew under the auspices of Narendra Nath but it was Girindrasekhar Bose who played a significant role in popularizing psychology and psychoanalysis. Bose was the first person to receive a doctorate in psychology from the University of Calcutta.[141] He published several articles on psychology and psychoanalysis and his contributions towards the development of psychology in India are enormous. Bose was not interested in the plain application of Western psychological concepts and techniques and felt that more research should be done on traditional Indian psychology.[142] Bose was the founder of the Indian Psychoanalytical Society established in 1922. He interacted with Sigmund Freud, Ernest Jones, and William A. White,

---

[138] Berkeley-Hill contributed a chapter, 'Importance of Mental Hygiene', on mental hygiene in Birendra Nath Ghosh, *A Treatise on Hygiene and Public Health: With Special Reference to the Tropics* (Calcutta: Scientific Publishing, 9th ed., 1938), 357.

[139] Hans Pols, '"Beyond the Clinical Frontier": The American Mental Hygiene Movement, 1910–1945', in *International Relations in Psychiatry: Britain, Germany, & The United States to World War II*, edited by Volker Roelcke, Paul J. Weindling, and Louise Westwood (Rochester: University of Rochester Press, 2010), 111.

[140] Nandy, *The Savage Freud and Other Essays*, 95.

[141] Hartnack, *Psychoanalysis in Colonial India*, 98.

[142] Hartnack, *Psychoanalysis in Colonial India*, 96.

all of whom appreciated his work. Psychoanalysis was systematically pursued by some British officials as well. Berkeley-Hill applied psychoanalytic theories on Indian patients. He published several papers analysing Indians habits, culture, and society.[143] Hartnack argues that Berkeley-Hill utilized psychoanalysis to criticize elements of Indian society and culture as this allowed him to justify British rule in India. Bose on the other hand criticized Western concepts of psychoanalysis and regarded them as inadequate in unravelling the Indian psyche. Thus, psychoanalysis was used by Indians and Europeans to both critique and justify British rule.[144] Ernst has recently observed that 'historians too have been much more fascinated by the development of psychoanalysis in India than by mainstream psychiatry ... all of which is far less exotic in appeal for social and cultural historians than engagement with the role of sexuality, the unconscious mind and mechanisms of repression in regard to individual, cultural and political processes'.[145] Historians have so far focused on psychoanalysis, while psychiatry remains a relatively unexplored area. But it should be kept in mind that psychology and psychoanalysis witnessed growth and institutionalization because they developed outside the control of the colonial state. Indians contributed to the growth and the development of these disciplines thereby benefitted Indians. Psychiatry on the other hand witnessed restricted growth due to the constraints of colonial control.

Peter Conrad and Joseph W. Schiender pointed out that 'a unitary, popular and finally dominant concept of mental illness developed only in the late eighteenth century. It was not an overnight revolution, but rather a gradual development over more than two centuries'.[146] By the twentieth century, they argued that the process of medicalization was complete. Dominance over the conception and treatment of madness had been achieved.[147] In other words, medicalization meant reification

[143] Hartnack, *Psychoanalysis in Colonial India*, 32–3.

[144] Hartnack, *Psychoanalysis in Colonial India*, 195.

[145] Waltraud Ernst, 'The Indianization of Colonial Medicine: The Case of Psychiatry in Early-Twentieth Century British India', *Journal of the History of Science, Technology and Medicine*, vol. 20, no. 4 (2012): 71.

[146] Peter Conrad and Joseph W. Schneider, *Deviance and Medicalization: From Badness to Sickness* (Philadelphia, Temple University Press, 1993), 47.

[147] Conrad and Schneider, *Deviance and Medicalization*, 71.

of the medical machinery, that is, science and technology were used to pathologize and prescribe the suitable cure for particular diseases. This process led to the objectification of humans by declaring them patients, giving complete control to doctors. However, medicalization of psychiatry in India was quite different than in the West. Here, it was the by-product of colonialism. There exist no clear antecedents from which one can draw any direct relationship between the 'indigenous' and 'Western' understanding of insanity and its cure. The psychiatric power and its claim to a superior cure of insanity drew authority from colonialism. Thus, the process of medicalization of psychiatry in colonial India should not be seen in unitary terms. The paraphernalia of psychiatric infrastructure had fully emerged by the twentieth century but the state refused to take responsibility of the mentally ill. The national movement was seen as an impediment. The government spent its energy to meet the immediate medical needs of the Indian population. But, it would not be inappropriate to argue that psychiatry remained at the margins of the medicinal interventions. Shruti Kapila argues that 'government prerogatives of both financial stringency and medical priorities overrode any comprehensive conception of a profession'.[148]

India still lacked a professional body of psychiatrists. There was no institution that could unite the psychiatrists as a group of individuals. Roger Jeffery argues that 'after 1922 a limit of one Indian to every two European recruits was set' for the IMS.[149] This indeed hastened the process of Indianization. After this period one does witness Indians being appointed to high posts such as that of the Superintendent of asylums. The first Indian Superintendent of the Agra Mental Hospital, Banarsi Das, played an important role in the establishment of a professional body. In Britain, the Royal Medico-Psychological Association was the main organization of psychiatry. Its origin dated back to 1841 when an 'Association of Medical Officers of Asylums and Hospitals' was formed. From 1866 to 1925 this body was known as the Medico-Psychological Association, and between 1926 and 1971 it was called the Royal Medico-Psychological Association. In 1971 a new charter was granted to the association whereby it was constituted as the Royal

---

[148] Kapila, 'The Making of Colonial Psychiatry', 98.
[149] Jeffery, 'Recognizing India's Doctors', 312.

College of Psychiatrists.[150] Initially the association met annually but after 1866 its meetings took place once in every quarter. The body had a professional journal in which its members published their research. After almost a hundred years of the founding of the Royal Medico-Psychological Association, an Indian Division came up in 1936, called the Royal Indian Medical Psychological Association.

Banarsi Das wrote letters requesting the Director General of the IMS to facilitate the functioning of the association. He pointed out that 'an Association could only function if local governments would provide leave and travelling allowance to its members for the annual meetings.'[151] After the formation of the Royal Indian Medical Psychological Association, the government conceded his demand and requested provincial governments to assist the members. J. A Thorne, Joint Secretary to the Government of India, stated in this context that 'the object of the Indian division is to encourage the study of mental diseases by means of periodical meetings at some central Mental Hospital which will provide an opportunity for alienists in India to pool their experiences and to exchange ideas on problems of psychiatry and administration of mental hospitals.'[152] The first meeting was held in 1939 at the Punjab Mental Hospital and it was attended by 24 members. Dr C. J. Thomas, member of the Royal Medico-Psychological Association, attended the meeting.[153]

In 1922, the Ranchi European Mental Hospital got affiliation from the University of London to start a diploma course in psychological

[150] Thomas Bewley, *Madness to Mental Illness: A History of the Royal College of Psychiatrists* (London: The Royal College of Psychiatrists, 2008), 2.

[151] Proposal to Form an Indian Division of the Royal Medico-Psychological Association and Grant Special Casual Leave and Travelling Expenses to Its Men for Attending the Annual Meetings of the Division at Some Mental Hospital in India, Home/Jails, File No. 128/36, 1936, NAI.

[152] Proposal to Form an Indian Division of the Royal Medico-Psychological Association and Grant Special Casual Leave and Travelling Expenses to Its Men for Attending the Annual Meetings of the Division at Some Mental Hospital in India, Home/Jails, File No. 128/36, 1936, NAI.

[153] Proposal to Form an Indian Division of the Royal Medico-Psychological Association and Grant Special Casual Leave and Travelling Expenses to Its Men for Attending the Annual Meetings of the Division at Some Mental Hospital in India, Home/Jails, File No. 128/36, 1936, NAI.

medicine.[154] A similar attempt was made in 1932 when mental nursing in India got recognition from St. Andrew's Hospital, Northampton.[155] These attempts were rather rare and they failed to alter the overall situation. A handful of Indians were sent abroad to study psychiatry. Banarsi Das published an article in 1931 about his psychiatric tour to Europe in that year. He wrote that 'through the generosity of the United Provinces Government, I undertook a tour of visits to some of the important mental institutions of Europe'.[156] He visited the Bethlem Royal Hospital at London, Craig House at Edinburgh (a private hospital), and a psychiatric clinic at The Hague in Holland, and psychiatric hospitals and clinics in Germany, Austria, and France, observing and learning about the advances made in psychiatry in these countries. Even on the eve of decolonization, therefore, Indians continued to travel to England, America, and Europe to gain experience and training given that psychiatric education in India lagged behind the West.

Professor Edward Mapother of the Maudsley Hospital, London, visited Sri Lanka (then Ceylon) and India in 1937. He made a damning critique of the overall psychiatric infrastructure while claiming that the British were 'bearing the white man's burden'.[157] Mapother regarded the psychiatric infrastructure as the white man's burden because he believed that the British were doing the best that was possible under the circumstances. He argued that 'it is probable that the situation would have been as bad under the rule of any European nation, and worse under the Indians themselves, but one cannot expect Indians to accept this argument as finality'.[158] He wrote that 'the wretched provision for the

[154] S. Haque Nizame and Nishant Goyal, 'History of Psychiatry in India', *Indian Journal of Psychiatry*, vol. 52, no. 7 (January 2010): 9.

[155] Enquiry as to the recognition in India of the Certificate in Mental Nursing by the Royal Medico-Psychological Association, St. Andrew Hospital, Northampton, Home/Jails, File No. 124, 1932, NAI.

[156] Banarsi Das, 'A Psychiatric Tour of Europe', *Indian Medical Gazette*, vol. 66, no. 9 (September 1931): 517–18.

[157] Papers of Edward Mapother, Treatment of Mental Disorder in India, EM-01, Royal Bethlem Hospital Archives (I owe this particular reference to Dr Alok Sarin).

[158] Papers of Edward Mapother, Treatment of Mental Disorder in India, EM-01, Royal Bethlem Hospital Archives.

insane in India is apt to be excused in particular by reference to the cost of other medical purposes.'[159] He attributed these pathetic conditions to overcrowding and lack of infrastructure. James H. Mills and Sanjeev Jain have analysed the Mapother Report and have pointed out that 'Mapother's visit in the decade before the end of Empire in South Asia provides an insight into the rather more complicated power relations of medicine in the period'. This period was marked by Indianization, which resulted in an intense struggle between Indians and Europeans.[160] Mapother noted,

> It is clear that in the future as never in the past, the progress of psychiatry in India will depend almost wholly upon those educated in India. The creation of an effective service of psychiatrists and the improvement of undergraduate and postgraduate training necessary for this seems bound to become business hereafter of the separate governments of each province or presidency.[161]

On the one hand he was aware of the necessity of the change, but on the other hand he remained doubtful about such transformation being achieved.

Mapother visited all the major psychiatric institutions of India. His report was not published and it was decided that the information obtained was for personal use and for preparing a report for the Government of Ceylon. For obvious reasons the report was suppressed as it would invite widespread criticism. Mapother held consultations with the President of the Medical Board and the Director General of Medical Service. Both were aware of the conspicuous lack of the psychiatric structure but it was clear that the Government was not prepared for massive modifications. The rising national movement and lack of funds were regarded as major impediments. It is evident that the colonial state

---

[159] Papers of Edward Mapother, Treatment of Mental Disorder in India, EM-01, Royal Bethlem Hospital Archives.

[160] James H. Mills and Sanjeev Jain, 'Mapother of the Maudsley and Psychiatry at the End of the Raj', in *Psychiatry and Empire*, edited by Sloan Mahone and Megan Vaughan (New York: Palgrave Macmillan: 2007), 155.

[161] Papers of Edward Mapother, Treatment of Mental Disorder in India, EM-01, Royal Bethlem Hospital Archives.

was washing its hands off the responsibilities as these liabilities had to be eventually borne by Indians. Mapother's assessments were confirmed by the Health Survey and Development Committee (1946), also known as the Bhore Committee after its Chairperson, Joseph Bhore.[162] The committee highlighted the appalling conditions of health services in India. Mental hospitals were also surveyed by Colonel M. Taylor, Medical Superintendent of the Ranchi European Mental Hospital. He pointed out that 'the majority of the Mental Hospitals in India are quite out of date, and are designed for detention and safe custody without regard to curative treatment. The worst of them—the Punjab Mental Hospital, the Thana Mental Hospital, the Agra Mental Hospital, and the Nagpur Mental Hospital favour of the Workhouse and the Prison, and should be rebuilt.'[163] He further argued that the Superintendents of six of these hospitals 'have little or no postgraduate experience or training in psychological medicine.'[164]

The Bhore Committee started surveying health services in 1943 and its final report was submitted in 1946. According to the report, the total accommodation available in 1946 for treatment of mental illness was 10,189 beds. It was noted that 'the functioning of existing mental institutions, in most cases, [was] far from satisfactory'. Although the committee had envisaged reform based on its recommendations to be instituted after World War II ended, by then the political turmoil in India was at its peak. It was only later that many of the recommendations of the Bhore Committee laid the basis of health reform in independent India.[165] On the other hand, after the death of Banarsi Das in 1943, Lieutenant Colonel Moore Taylor, the Superintendent of the European Mental Hospital at Ranchi, took over the presidentship of the Indian division of the Royal Medico-Psychological Association. By this time World War II and the nationalist upsurge were already underway. In 1946 Moore Taylor's initiatives were directed towards the establishment of a separate Indian psychiatric society. In April 1947,

[162] Report of the Health Survey and Development Committee, vols I and II (Delhi: Manager of Publication, 1946).

[163] Report of the Health Survey and Development Committee, vol. 1, 131.

[164] Report of the Health Survey and Development Committee, vol. 1, 131.

[165] Report of the Health Survey and Development Committee, vol. 1, 131.

Taylor resigned as he felt that the Indian division was being allowed to die.[166] The new body was named as the Indian Psychiatric Society. Today it is the chief professional body of psychiatrists in India. The state often supported such initiatives because India did not have specialist facilities for training and education. Up till the late 1950s majority of psychiatrists were sent abroad for training. The Bhore Committee recommended the creation of the All India Institute of Mental Health, which was established in Bangalore with the aim of providing postgraduate training in psychiatry, clinical psychology, and for conducting research in mental health. Later, in 1962, the institute was renamed as the National Institute of Mental Health and Neurosciences.[167] E. A. Bennet, the senior physician in psychotherapy in Maudsley hospital and consulting psychiatrist, remarked,

> Mechanical restraint was routine in some of provincial civil mental hospitals as recently as 1945 and even shackles, chains and hand cuffs, while unusual, were by no means unknown ... The Punjab Mental Hospital in Lahore (800 bed) contains some well-designed modern wards. The two hospitals at Ranchi and the Mysore state hospital, near Bangalore, stand out as two examples of what may be achieved elsewhere.[168]

***

The chapter makes it amply clear that the colonial state remained indifferent towards the mentally ill throughout the period. We can gauge this primarily from the plethora of reports examined above that the state was apathetic to the insane incarcerated in asylums. It should be noted that by and large 'harmless' lunatics were considered to be a burden by the state but the practice of incarcerating them was generally discouraged.

It also demonstrates that mid-twentieth century onwards few medical men made major contributions towards transforming the nature

---

[166] Sanjeev Jain, 'Psychiatry and Confinement in India', in *The Confinement of Insane: International Perspectives 1800–1965*, edited by Roy Porter and David Wright (Cambridge: Cambridge University Press, 2003), 293.

[167] Ratna Verma, *Psychiatric Social Work in India* (New Delhi: Sage, 1991), 47.

[168] E. A. Bennet, 'Psychiatry in India and Pakistan', *The Indian Journal of Neurology and Psychiatry*, vol. 1, no. 1 (January–March 1949): 36.

of psychiatry in India. Wider exposure to international trends was an important feature of twentieth-century psychiatry in India. These men not only travelled widely but also experimented with new methods of treatment, as we saw in the case of psychoanalysis and the mental hygiene movement. However, as these efforts were frequently confined to individuals, they cannot be generalized.

The chapter also highlights the significance of the reform cycle triggered as a direct consequence of the IHDC's report. Reorganization was initiated not because of the colonial state's intention to reform, but instead in an attempt to redirect the energies and attention of critics of colonial drug policies at both the national and international levels towards something more palpable. The colonial state also ensured the continuous supply of revenue from hemp cultivation. The result was shoddy reorganization that had short-term gains, with the restructuring of asylum management becoming redundant in a decade or two since the IHDC reforms. India had mammoth asylums but lacked the facilities and infrastructure required for their management.

Here it has also been argued that in colonial north India, psychiatrists felt the need of modernization more than any other group. The emergence of the figure of a 'psychiatrist' was an unintended consequence of the aforesaid reform. This consolidation of the psychiatrist's identity was further connected to multiple processes that included administrative reforms, legislative changes, epistemological shifts, and political alterations at both the national and international levels. Psychiatrists such as Charles Lodge Patch, W. S. J. Shaw, Berkeley-Hill, and Banarsi Das, to name a few, began to play a crucial role in the modernization of their profession. In fact, it may be argued that the second wave of reform that started from the second decade of the twentieth century was more a result of individual efforts. These changes were neither unilinear nor inevitably productive but instead reflected the tumultuous path of modernization.

Legislative reform and medical advancement at least theoretically also made 'curative treatment' an essential part of the mental hospitals. The 1912 Act furthered the practice of class-based treatment since it made the admission process lengthy and expensive. The mental hospital no longer remained an abode for the poor as they used to be in the nineteenth century. Indians were given treatment in some of these hospitals according to their economic status. Wealthy Indians had access to first-class treatment in some of the mental hospitals by the twentieth century. Bhattacharyya has erroneously argued that 'with the rise of the psychiatric expert and the increasingly significant role of medical education in India, the asylum was transformed into a singularly colonial and homogeneous space'.[169] This chapter on the other hand shows that while some of the mental hospitals witnessed advancement, others continued to exist as mere receptacles of the mentally ill. The zeal of the respective Superintendents was an important factor that determined whether an institution was to be a lunatic asylums or mental hospital. It has also demonstrated how colonial modernity with its ambiguities attempted to allocate the burden on the 'natives' by only *attempting* to provide (in)adequate psychiatric infrastructure, without actually delivering on the promise. The result of this superficial modernization was that India never had facilities for those who wanted to become specialists, and even after several of the reforms, anyone who desired to specialize in psychiatry had to go to Britain. This sort of dependency fettered the development of modern psychiatry in India.

---

[169] Bhattacharyya, 'Indian Insanes', iv.

2 Managing Madness

Architecture, Medicine, and Personnel

> In India up to now the asylums have been built on prison lines, and though the underground dungeons at Bhowanipore have not been used for many years, the modern cells, though larger, airier and above ground, are of the same type.[1]

Lunatic asylums, largely 'custodial' in nature, were complex hierarchical structures that preserved hierarchies between the 'sane' and the 'insane', 'white' and 'black', and 'high' and 'low' castes and classes. These binaries were an intrinsic part of colonial medicine. The 'insane hospitals' were renamed 'mental hospitals' by the second decade of the twentieth century, and this chapter maps the changes that took place in terms of architecture, medicine, and treatment in these institutions. The novel

---

[1] Plans for the New Central Asylum to Be Constructed at Lahore, Home Dept/ Medical Branch Nos 66 to 85, May 1899, NAI.

principles of moral management became obsolete as the fears of degeneration gave psychiatry a biological turn. Not only did the architectural values change but the underlying 'scientific' understanding of madness, its diagnosis, and treatment underwent fundamental transformations. This chapter examines the ways in which bureaucratic experiences were structured, organized, and reified into modern Indian psychiatry.

Space, Place, and Architecture

Nineteenth-century 'asylum science' laid enormous emphasis on the architecture of the asylum. These asylums, it may be mentioned, were usually located away from urban areas. The curable had to be separated from the 'incurables', the 'violent' from the 'harmless', and the 'epileptic' from the 'idiots' for the effective management of the asylums. High principles related to such moral architecture were constantly considered but were not regarded practical enough to be executed. The reason offered behind this failed ideal was financial stringency and it was also argued that racial difference required divergent measures. Asylum architecture in India remained archaic and was based on the notions of prison architecture.

Insane asylums were established in colonial India towards the end of the eighteenth century. The colonial government was reluctant to establish asylum buildings during the first half of the nineteenth century. There existed a continuous use of other buildings such as jails and dispensaries to incarcerate insane 'natives'.[2] These provisions were made to economize living costs. Only in the latter half of the nineteenth century were more built structures turned into lunatic asylums. Biswamoy Pati attempted to untangle the conspicuous relationship between the Cuttack Lunatic Asylum and the jail. He argued:

> In fact, this implied the rather predictable expansion of the Cuttack Jail to accommodate the Lunatic Asylum, with the latter developing as it were from 'within the womb' of the Cuttack Jail. Though we are not told anything about the labour obtained for this purpose it would be difficult to

[2] Some of the earliest references regarding the establishment of the native insane asylum are available in the Bengal despatches. These files reveal government intent to establish separate asylums for the 'natives' as they found it inconvenient to incarcerate the insane in jails.

imagine that the inmates of the Jail (viz. which included the prisoners and the 'criminal' lunatics—if not only the 'lunatics') were not involved with the construction of the Asylum.[3]

Asylums throughout the nineteenth century, it may be argued, continued to thrive and survive as part of the prison structures. Asylums were planned in such a way that the jail's proximity could be assured, which helped shift 'criminal' lunatics from one place to another and borrow instruments of correction when required. The nearness of prisons also left an indelible mark on asylum architecture since throughout the nineteenth and the first half of the twentieth centuries asylum buildings were regarded as 'glorified prisons'.

The Delhi Asylum was situated outside the walls of the city of Delhi, near the Delhi Gate and about 200 yards away from the Delhi Jail. It may be noted that according to the Delhi State Gazetteer, the lunatic asylum was founded in 1840.[4] This asylum was sacked on 11 May 1857 and all the 110 inmates escaped.[5] After the 1857 Rebellion, the asylum was again reorganized and continued to function till 1861. Thereafter, the inmates were transferred to the Lahore asylum, and the building was used as a workshop of the Delhi jail. The Delhi asylum was re-established in 1867 due to the significant efforts of the Civil Surgeon of Delhi, Dr J. C. Penny.[6] The government was reluctant, however, to establish an asylum in Delhi. It was argued that even though

there is at present but one lunatic asylum in the Punjab, at Lahore ... [it] by no means follows that Delhi is the best place for an additional asylum.

[3] Biswamoy Pati, 'Confining "Lunatics": The Cuttack Asylum, c. 1864–1906', in *Society, Medicine and Politics in Colonial India*, edited by Biswamoy Pati and Mark Harrison (New York: Routledge, 2018).

[4] Gazetteer of the Delhi District, 1883–84, Compiled and Published under the authority of Punjab Government, 156. The records of the Delhi asylum before 1861 are difficult to locate.

[5] The Annual Reports of the Lunatic Asylums of the Punjab for the year 1871, NAI. New research has revealed that all inmates of the Delhi asylum did not escape during the revolt of 1857. The asylum continued to provide shelter to some of the insane. For details, see Mahmood Farooqui, *Besieged: Voices from Delhi 1857* (Delhi: Penguin, 2010).

[6] Gazetteer of the Delhi District, 1883–84, 156.

It is not central, not very healthy; again it is on extremity of Punjab, and in several respects particularly unhealthy—fevers and virulent ulcers being often epidemic here. If a second asylum be eventually founded, probably Umballah would be better place.[7]

Subsequently, however, the Delhi asylum was permanently closed and 1 March 1900 onwards a new asylum at Lahore had been established and all the patients—103 males and 35 females—of the Delhi asylum were transferred to the new Lahore asylum on 23 March 1900.[8] Henceforth, the Punjab only had one central lunatic asylum, the Lahore Lunatic Asylum.

In the case of the Delhi asylum, a map before the revolt of 1857 shows that it was situated outside the walled city of Delhi—it was built opposite to the jail (see Figure 2.1). It is pertinent that, according to Foucault, 'it was this separation and confinement that hid away unreason, and betrayed the shame it aroused; but it explicitly drew attention to madness and pointed towards it.'[9] However, there were notions other than those associated with the stigmatization of madness that played a role in the location of the asylums at a distance from the urban centres. Lunatics were considered to be dangerous and senseless. Their insanity deprived them of their senses and thus they forgot the essential difference between 'black' and 'white'. The asylum was to be located far away from European habitation as the appearance of the 'filthy' and 'naked' insane on the streets or in close proximity to Europeans was disturbing. Waltraud Ernst has analysed the issue of space in the context of colonial India and she situates 'space' both at the 'ideological and geographical' levels. Her work points out 'how distance between different classes and races were maintained by means of geographical separation (namely the deportation of insane Europeans back to Europe); and extra institutional segregation (i.e. the establishment of separate asylums in

[7] Re-establishment of the Delhi Asylum, Home Dept./Public Branch, Proceedings A., File No. 70–71, 25 October 1865, NAI.

[8] The Annual Report of the Lunatic Asylum of the Punjab for the Year 1900, National Medical Library.

[9] Michel Foucault, *Madness and Civilization: A History of Insanity in the Age of Reason*, translated by Richard Howard (London: Routledge, 2001), 65.

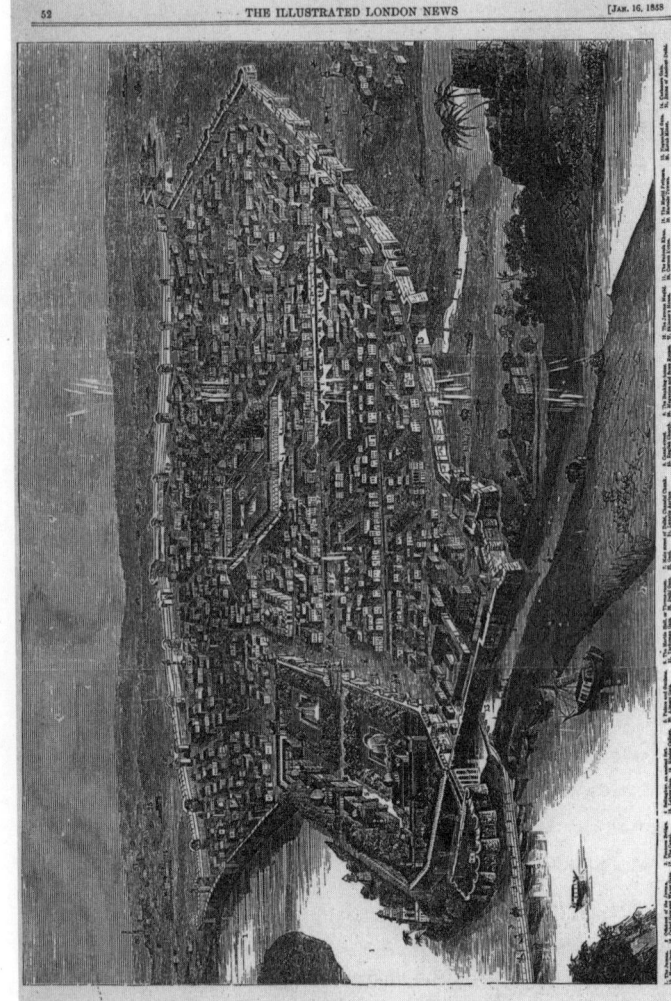

THE CITY OF DELHI BEFORE THE SIEGE.

Figure 2.1   The city of Delhi before the Revolt of 1857. No. 21: lunatic asylum

Source: The Illustrated London News, 1858.

India, for "natives" on the one hand and Europeans waiting repatriation on the other)".[10]

Throughout the period, Delhi was considered to be an unsuitable place for the establishment of the lunatic asylum. Innumerable plans were discussed to shift the asylum from Delhi to Meerut.[11] However, these plans never materialized. Agra was also considered to be a suitable place for the establishment of an asylum for 'native' lunatics. George Cowper Barnet, Secretary to the Government of North-western Frontier Provinces, writing to the Government of India declared, 'it is not so distant from Ajmere, or from the district of the Jhansie Division ... the climate is believed to be congenial to the native constitution'.[12] Agra was regarded as an unhealthy location as far the European constitution was concerned. At the time of the reorganization of the lunatic asylums in 1897, it was suggested that 'an asylum for European and Eurasian inmates be established at Nasik'.[13] However, plans for the construction of an asylum at Nasik were abandoned and a central asylum for the European patients was set up at Ranchi in 1918.

Notions of medical topography revolved around European bodily constitutions. While the constitution of the 'native' was taken into consideration, priority was given either to strategic locations or on the basis of European requirements. Mark Harrison argues that the mapping of India's climatic zones was similar to that of the botanical and military topographic surveys conducted in the eighteenth century. He asserts that this process known as 'medical topography' led to the categorization of climatic zones as healthy or unhealthy in the nineteenth century. These ideas influenced views regarding the well-being of the superior

---

[10] Waltraud Ernst, 'Madness and Colonial Spaces—British India, c. 1800–1947', in *Madness, Architecture and the Built Environment*, edited by Leslie Topp, James E. Moran, and Jonathan Andrews (London: Routledge, 2007), 216.

[11] The Annual Return of the Insane Hospitals at Delhi, Bareilly and Baneres for the year 1853, E/4/ 833, British Library (BL).

[12] Proposal for the Construction for the Lunatic Asylum at Agra, Home Dept./Public Branch, File No. 26 to 30, 20 October 1862, NAI.

[13] Proposed Improvement in the Administration of Lunatic Asylum in India, Home Dept./Medical Branch, File No. 97–99, March 1895, NAI.

race prevalent in Anglo-Indian medicine.[14] A number of sites for the construction of asylums were at times chosen and then abandoned as they were regarded as unsuitable in terms of 'medical topography'. A latent underlying motive behind the abandonment of several asylum sites was government apathy towards mental illness. It has been argued elsewhere that 'built space was an important part of colonial psychiatry', which is indicated by the fact that considerable details related to asylum architecture were provided in the James Clark Enquiry. The questions formulated by the enquiry such as 'Were these [buildings] originally designed for a lunatic asylum? Do they form a part of other buildings such as hospital, prisons, & etc.?'[15] shows the fact that the government consciously approved structures originally built for other purposes to be appropriated for use as asylums. Only 'fifty percent of the buildings were purpose-built as asylums, the rest were older structures that were converted into asylums. Seventy percent of these second-hand structures had formed a part of buildings such as jails—a clear pointer towards their being perceived of as punitive spaces.'[16] This conversion of other institutions such as hospitals and prisons, mostly the latter, to asylums also points to the lack of the colonial government's commitment to public health broadly and particularly to problems of 'mental health' of the subject population, which can be attributed to factors as narrow as financial stringency. Debjani Das also points out that 'throughout the nineteenth century, asylum buildings were built and rebuilt. At times, the site of the asylum was changed, and other times, extensions were made to the existing building'.[17]

The Lahore asylum also witnessed several relocations: The Transylvanian physician of Maharaja Daleep Singh, Dr Johann Martin Honigberger, kept in his custody 12 lunatics.[18] After the annexation

[14] Mark Harrison, *Climates and Constitutions: Health, Race, Environment and British Imperialism in India 1600–1850* (New Delhi: Oxford University Press, 1999), 114.

[15] Sir James Clark's Enquiry as to the Care and the Treatment of Lunatics, Home Dept./Public Branch, File Nos 22–3, 19 December 1868, NAI.

[16] Shilpi Rajpal, 'Colonial Psychiatry in Mid-Nineteenth Century India: The James Clark Enquiry', *South Asia Research*, vol. 35, no. 1 (2015): 72.

[17] Debjani Das, *Houses of Madness: Insanity and Asylums of Bengal in Nineteenth Century India* (New Delhi: Oxford University Press, 2015), 55.

[18] Charles J. Lodge Patch, *A Critical Review of the Punjab Mental Hospitals from 1840–1930* (Lahore Record Office: Punjab Government, 1931), 1.

of the Punjab in 1849, these lunatics were handed over to Dr Hathaway, who confined them to a stable. Their number went up to 85 within the next 10 years.[19] It was only after the 1857 Rebellion that an asylum was established near the Anarkali Bazaar of the city.[20] This asylum was later shifted to Lehna Singh's Chownee in 1868.[21] At the beginning of the twentieth century, the asylum was again relocated, this time outside the city near the Lahore Jail.[22]

The Lahore asylum was the first to be centralized following the reform and reorganization that occurred along the lines of the recommendation of the IHDC. The architectural planning of the asylum created much confusion in official circles. The more liberal-minded officials wished to create a modern asylum based on the European style. An unofficial memorandum drawn up by the Director General of Medicine, Robert Harvey, was placed before the British Indian Government, where it was noted,

> In India up to now the asylums have been built on prison lines, and though the underground dungeons at Bhowanipore have not been used for many years, the modern cells, though larger, airier and above ground, are of the same type. Solitary confinement, as is well known, is so severe a punishment that the law limits its duration. Yet in most Indian asylum the greater part of lunatics are kept in solitary cells, at all events at night. ... I have today visited the old, and the site for the new, asylum at Lahore. The old one is a serai adapted for the purposes of the safe keeping of lunatics on strict prison lines ... The new asylum, though it will be a great improvement on the old one, is planned on the same lines and will be nothing more than a somewhat glorified prison in [sic] by a containing wall 15 feet high with a second wall also 15 feet high round the yard for non-criminals.[23]

W. M. Young, the Lieutenant Governor of Punjab, wrote a personal note to the Secretary to the Lieutenant Gogvernor of Punjab, C. M. Rivaz,

[19] Patch, *A Critical Review of the Punjab Mental Hospitals*, 10.

[20] Patch, *A Critical Review of the Punjab Mental Hospitals*, 17.

[21] Patch, *A Critical Review of the Punjab Mental Hospitals*, 23.

[22] Patch, *A Critical Review of the Punjab Mental Hospitals*, 23.

[23] Plans for the New Central Asylum to Be Constructed at Lahore, Home Dept/Medical Branch, Nos 66 to 85, May 1899, NAI.

in which he not only mocked Harvey's suggestion but also pointed out that 'Harvey's mild lunatics are at large and are to be met all over the province'.[24] He further pointed out that 'the people whom we put under restraint are mostly either dangerous or offensive, and one of our objects is attention to therapeutics and another humane treatment, I can't agree to 500 mad people, many of them violent, being turned loose in Lahore'.[25] He further asserted, 'Personally, I think the note had better been pigeonholed for good'.[26] These racialized remarks point towards the prejudice of considering the entire subject population as 'irrational'. Racial remarks permeated the writings of British officials, who justified the existence and continuation of empire. Asylums necessarily were part of penalizing structures. Words such as 'offensive', 'dangerous', or 'wild' should be seen as semiotics of British policies that reflect issues of governance inside and outside the asylums.

James Moran and Leslie Topp have argued that 'the key importance of spatial separation to the history of psychiatry, space and architecture has arguably been emphasized even more by psychiatrists, architects, reformers others than they have by those dedicated to the wider field of medicine'.[27] The preceding discussion reflects that racial separation should be regarded as a 'hallmark' of the colonial asylum architecture. Harvey also suggested that high walls be replaced by cactus hedges. In his words, 'A wall is necessary for a criminal yard, although with careful supervision breaking out of the wards should be impossible. Another may be required round the enclosure of the women, but in both cases an iron railing which would allow circulation of air should be substituted for the proposed mud walls'.[28] H. J. Maynard in the same letter had

---

[24] Plans for the New Central Asylum to Be Constructed at Lahore, Home Dept/Medical Branch, Nos 66 to 85, May 1899, NAI.

[25] Plans for the New Central Asylum to Be Constructed at Lahore, Home Dept/Medical Branch, Nos 66 to 85, May 1899, NAI.

[26] Plans for the New Central Asylum to Be Constructed at Lahore, Home Dept/Medical Branch, Nos 66 to 85, May 1899, NAI.

[27] James Moran and Leslie Topp, 'Introduction: Interpreting Psychiatric Spaces', in Madness, Architecture and the Built Environment, edited by Leslie Topp, James E. Moran, and Jonathan Andrews (London: Routledge, 2007), 1.

[28] Moran and Topp, 'Introduction', 1.

countered Harvey's viewpoint by pointing out the differences in the ways of life that prevailed in Europe and in the Punjab province respectively. Maynard stated,

> In a Punjab village both in summer and winter the people, when not at work in their fields, live habitually within walls and ordinarily every native house is a walled enclosure without ventilation or windows. Apart, therefore, from the special considerations which apply to the case of the women, owing to the widespread idea of the propriety of 'purdah', it is probable that a native of the Punjab finds a walled enclosure more congenial to his habits and comfortable than an open compound.[29]

Such a justification can only be understood in terms of the logics of colonial policies that discriminated against certain communities.[30] It can be regarded as a logic of colonial governance that sanctioned a continuation of 'native practice' thereby concealing its violence. Therefore, a 'native' of the Punjab was used to being within walls.

Lunatics in India could not be compared to lunatics in Europe or elsewhere as the so-called Indian brand of lunatics was considered to be 'dangerous' and 'offensive'. They could not be 'let loose' or 'cured properly' and thus they had to be incarcerated. W. M. Young's views were commonly prevalent and had general acceptance during the period. A conference was called upon to consider the issues raised by Director General Harvey. The Lahore asylum was proposed to be constructed on the panopticon model of Bentham (see Figure 2.2).[31] Ganga Ram, who

[29] Moran and Topp, 'Introduction', 1.

[30] The colonial state typified certain communities as 'manly' while others they labelled as effeminate. As it has been discussed, Punjabis were regarded as 'manly' and 'violent', while Bengalis were regarded as effeminate. For details, see Mrinalini Sinha, *Colonial Masculinity: The 'Manly Englishman' and the 'Effeminate Bengali' in the Late Nineteenth Century* (Manchester: Manchester University Press, 1995). Further, other communities and certain tribes were rendered as criminals. For details, see Meena Radhakrishna, *Dishonoured by History: 'Criminal Tribes' and British Colonial Policy* (Delhi: Orient Blackswan, 2001).

[31] Jeremy Bentham was an English philosopher and jurist (1748–1832). His ideas about the panopticon structure of buildings were widely adapted in nineteenth-century England. The panopticon structure consists of round

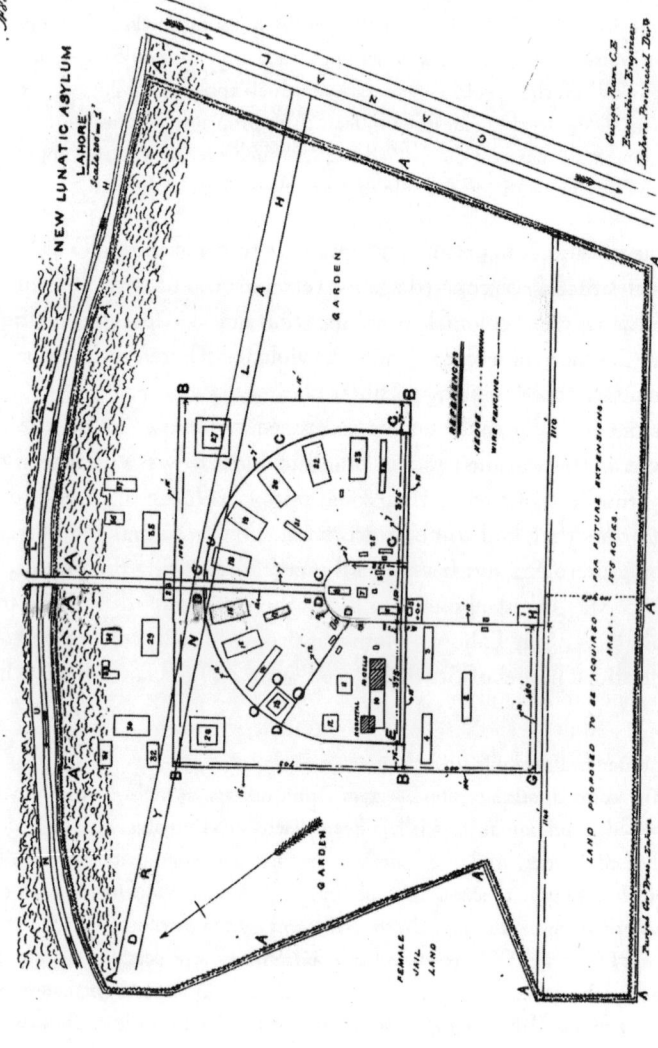

Figure 2.2 Plan for the Lahore Lunatic Asylum
Source: Home Dept/Medical Branch, Nos 66 to 85, May 1899, NAI.

was at this time the most important architect in the city of Lahore, was the chief engineer of the lunatic asylum. He was also the chief architect of all the important buildings in colonial Lahore,[32] and was given the title of Rai Bahadur and later honoured with a knighthood.

Ten members were present at the conference, including the Inspector General(s) of Prisons and Hospitals, besides Ganga Ram. The conference was prefaced by 'its cordial sympathy with principle advocated by Surgeon Major General Harvey of substituting supervision for restraint in the management of lunatics, and its full acceptance of the view that this ideal is one to be worked up to in so far as circumstances allow.'[33]

Harvey's ideals were regarded with some favour but were considered impractical. H. J. Maynard, Judicial and General Secretary to the Government wrote in a letter to the Secretary to the Government of India: 'It is not the practice of the people of the Punjab to send their mild lunatics and harmless imbeciles to public asylums ... the vast majority of those confined in the asylums are either committed thither under the provisions of the Criminal Procedure Code or are persons "believed to be dangerous by the reasons of lunacy".'[34] The question of restraint was discussed at the conference in detail. It was stated that a 'fence and hedge would not prevent lunatics from escaping.'[35] Cactus hedge and iron railing were considered unsuitable and insecure. Further, the conference

---

buildings with a tower in between. The guard in the tower could observe patients/prisoners/officers in the cells. Michel Foucault discusses in his work *Discipline and Punish* the role that the panopticon played in facilitating surveillance. He argued that the panopticon was actually a laboratory of power since observance enabled dominance and control. For details, see Michel Foucault, *Discipline and Punish: The Birth of Prison*, translated by Alan Sheridan (New York: Vintage Book, 1995).

[32] A brief biographical sketch of Sir Ganga Ram is given in William J. Glover, *Making Lahore Modern: Constructing and Imagining a Colonial City* (Minneapolis: University of Minnesota Press, 2008), 84–5.

[33] Plans for the New Central Asylum to Be Constructed at Lahore, Home Dept/Medical Branch, Nos 66 to 85, May 1899, NAI.

[34] Plans for the New Central Asylum to Be Constructed at Lahore, Home Dept/Medical Branch, Nos 66 to 85, May 1899, NAI.

[35] Plans for the New Central Asylum to Be Constructed at Lahore, Home Dept./Medical Branch, Nos 66 to 85, May 1899, NAI.

considered reducing the height of asylum boundary walls from 15 feet to 12 feet.[36] Besides, issues related to recreation for and supervision of inmates were also discussed. Harvey believed that strict supervision was the best substitute for restraint. He had firm faith in the ideals of moral management. The delegates expressed general approval for such well-intentioned proposals but argued that an agency capable of exercising the moral influence required in order to give effect to the European method of treatment is not obtainable in the Punjab ... natives of the classes which accept work of this order have not the character or capacity which are required.[37] The issue of recreation was dealt with in a similar manner. The members attending the conference felt that the work-sheds in the asylums could be used for recreation and the day rooms requested by Surgeon General Harvey for the purpose were a matter left to the discretion of the respective whole-time Superintendents. These racialized arguments regarding lack of innate capacity of the 'natives' to be cured through therapeutics of moral management made them irremediable patients.

In 1922, a letter addressed to the editor was published in *The Statesman*, written by J. V. Jameson, a member of European associations, who highlighted the defects of the new European asylum built in Ranchi, which was supposed to have been built along the most up-to-date principles. Jameson wrote:

> The first impression that the visitor feels at entering the large blank gates is that he is entering a jail. This impression is heightened by the bareness of the building, lack of furniture, and other comforts of life which are to be found in every hospital. It is to be wondered at that a man accustomed to the ordinary amenities and comforts of life, whose brain being affected by illness or accident, should imagine that he has been put into jail for some unknown offence, when he finds himself confined in a small grey prison cell.[38]

[36] Plans for the New Central Asylum to Be Constructed at Lahore, Home Dept./Medical Branch, Nos 66 to 85, May 1899, NAI.

[37] Plans for the New Central Asylum to Be Constructed at Lahore, Home Dept./Medical Branch, Nos 66 to 85, May 1899, NAI.

[38] Amendment of the Indian Lunacy Act (IV of 1912), so as to provide the change of designation of lunatic asylums to mental hospitals, Home Dept./Jail Branch, File No. 88, 1922, NAI.

The architecture of asylum structures in India resembled that of prisons. Ideals were spoken about but were considered impractical. Historians working on the architecture of the colonial asylum have pointed out that asylum architecture of the metropolis when transferred to the colonies was largely out of date.[39] Outmoded Western architectural principles were often used but attempts were rarely made to indigenize and integrate local styles. Asylums, therefore, remained peripheral to the Indian imagination. While dispensaries, hospitals, and biomedicine were eventually integrated in the 'native' discourses of medicine and cure, *pagal khanas* or lunatic asylums due to their resemblance to prisons were unpopular and unacceptable by most of the Indian population up till the end of the colonial period.

The colonial state did not waste much energy or resources on the comfort of the inmates. Moreover, the question of space that was to be allotted to each patient remained unresolved throughout the nineteenth century. James Wise, the Superintendent in Charge of the Dacca asylum, remarked:

> The criminal population gets by the rule 54 superficial feet a man; the sepoy in the hospital is accommodated with 99 superficial feet; but up to the present time the case of the lunatic has not been considered; and the space which can be given to him is so limited.[40]

Wise argued that 54 'superficial' feet was insufficient for lunatics. But in the Cuttack asylum a lunatic was cramped within a space of 47 'superficial' feet.[41] In 1925, W. S. Jagoe Shaw, the Superintendent of the Central Institute for Mental Diseases at Yeravda, argued that 'a "dormitory" should give for each inmate 65 sq. feet of space and as a rule the ideal population be 16'.[42] Anil Persaud has discussed the issue

[39] Elizabeth Malcolm, 'Australian Asylum Architecture through German Eyes: Kew, Melbourne, 1867', *Health and History*, vol. 11, no. 1 (2009): 59–60.

[40] Sir James Clark's Enquiry as to the Care and the Treatment of Lunatics, Home Dept./Public Branch, File No. 22–23, 19 December 1868, NAI.

[41] Sir James Clark's Enquiry as to the Care and the Treatment of Lunatics, Home Dept./Public Branch, File No. 22–23, 19 December 1868, NAI.

[42] W. S. Jagoe Shaw, *A Clinical Handbook of Mental Diseases: For the Use of Students and Medical Practitioners in India* (Calcutta: Butterworth & Co., 1925), Appendix, p. viii.

of space on the ships transporting indentured labour from India to overseas colonies such as Guyana during the nineteenth century. He has pointed out that the "'superficial" space allotted to each adult [on the ship] was six feet by two feet.[43] Actually, however, 'the superficial space would have shrunk to 5.5 feet by 1.3 feet.'[44] In a similar manner, 65 sq ft was an ideal estimation but by the twentieth century, asylums were overcrowded and it would rarely have been the actual case that 65 sq ft of space could have been allotted to individual patients. In the twentieth century, the central asylum generally had around a thousand patients. There were separate infirmary and tubercle wards for sick patients. The solitary cells were for the 'most dangerous' class of patients. The criminal block was a walled area. The block for 'acute patients' was separate from that for 'chronic patients'. The administrative section had the office of the Superintendent and the clerical office. The bungalow of the Superintendent and the staff quarters were usually built within the hospital compound.

The basic conception underlying the asylum architectural design, namely that of a 'glorified' prison, remained an unquestionable reality of the mental hospitals in colonial India. Lofty ideals related to planning and designing were voiced as platitudes but, in practice, such high standards were never implemented. The basic principles of colonial architecture were 'segregation', 'order', and 'punishment'. The rhetoric of reform was continuously deployed to show the benevolent side of the Raj. The architectural norms that were declared redundant at home continued to be practised in the colonies. Notions about comfort and care were sidelined as the primary concern was related to the confinement of the 'dangerous' lunatics. Asylums were not designed to accommodate Indian needs and practices, and Western models were implemented without any concern for 'native' environmental and bodily requirements. Moreover, the strategic placement of mental hospitals outside city limits should be seen as a marker of racial discrimination that implied spatial

[43] Anil Persaud, 'Transformed Over Seas: "Medical Comforts" Aboard Nineteenth-Century Emigrant Ships', in *Labour Matters: Towards Global Histories*, edited by Marcel van der Linden and Prabhu P. Mahopatra (New Delhi: Tulika Books, 2009), 47.

[44] Persaud, 'Transformed Over Seas', 47.

segregation, the separation of 'white' from 'black' town. In this sense, the lunatics of the 'black town' were a double threat as they bypassed this divided line and had to be re-located through a double distancing—from the 'civilized white' as well as from the 'uncivilized natives'. The confinement of insanity within the asylum walls, one could say, ensured the safety and security of the British Raj.

The Professional Apparatus

The Superintendent was the head of an asylum. Throughout the nineteenth century, the Civil Surgeon of the area in which the respective asylums were located functioned as their Superintendents. They had to supervise an array of institutions such as jails, hospitals, asylums, and dispensaries. In spite of other duties, the Superintendents were expected to give 'full attention to the insane hospital under their charge, but also to entertain correct and enlighten views as to the proper mode of managing them [*sic*]'.[45] It was only from 1900 onwards that full-time Superintendents began to be specifically appointed to head the central asylums.[46] The moral management system considered the Superintendent as a father figure whose paternal affection and authority were essential for the treatment of those whose 'mind had gone astray'. Therefore, the Sperintendent's zeal for reform and his notions about madness, diagnosis, and treatment were critical for everyday governance. He often shaped the understanding and experiences of the staff and the inmates. The Superintendent's ideas were, therefore, important in shaping the management of the mental institution and treatment of the inmates.

The Annual Report of the Delhi Lunatic Asylum for the year 1871 tells us about Dr Penny's views which regarded insanity as being caused due to the consumption of intoxicants. He described in detail the ways

[45] Court despatch relating to the results of treatment of the inmates at the insane hospitals of Bareilly, Benares, and Delhi for the years 1846, 1847, and 1848, E/4/828, NAI.

[46] Scheme of Administration of Lunatic Asylums in India, and the Appointment of Whole-Time Superintendents to the Charge of Central Asylums, Home Depot/Medical Branch, Nos 54–71, March 1900, NAI.

in which Indian hemp was consumed and its harmful effects on the Indian population:

> In my small lunatic asylum in Delhi, during the past five years, I have had about 50 genuine well marked cases of mental disorder from the excessive use of Indian Hemp ... in the large city of Delhi where there are two lakhs of people, and especially amongst the Hindu population in excess of Mohammedans. Both the rich and poor amongst Hindus indulge in this narcotic, where the lowest classes of Mohammedans partake of it ... The habitual indulgers are to be found amongst saises, dhobi, faqueers, labourers, kahars, halalkhors ... After the stage of excitement the mind becomes confused, attention is arrested, man is stupid, and at last complete intoxication, in fact, it is the stage of depression.[47]

Penny was interested not only in the connection between hemp and insanity but also in the ways the general population used drugs. Scholars have pointed out that asylums were also places where knowledge was generated about local communities.[48] This knowledge helped in better governance of the unruly population. Penny played the model role of a colonial official who meticulously observed local practices helping in identifying and weeding out the 'troubled elements' of society. His successor, Dr Fairweather, successfully introduced practices of employment and manufacture in the Delhi asylum. The land near the lunatic asylum was reclaimed and a variety of new crops were grown.[49] Sarah Ann Pinto has argued that the Superintendents played a key role in maintaining order, generating knowledge about insanity, and ensuring productivity of the inmates.[50] Ernst's assessment that the Superintendents were

---

[47] The Annual Report of the Lunatic Asylums of the Punjab for the Year 1871, NAI.

[48] For discussion on knowledge production in the asylums, see James H. Mills, *Madness, Cannabis and Colonialism: The 'Native-Only' Lunatic Asylums of British India, 1857–1900* (Basingstoke: Macmillan, 2000); Sarah Ann Pinto, 'Shackled Bodies, Unchained Minds: Lunatic Asylums in Bombay Presidency, 1793–1921', unpublished PhD thesis, Victoria University of Wellington, 2017.

[49] The Annual Report of the Lunatic Asylums of the Punjab for the Year 1879, NAI.

[50] Pinto, 'Shackled Bodies, Unchained Minds', 61.

mere 'figureheads'[51] fails to carefully examine the significant role that the they played in shaping the institution. He had enormous power which was bestowed on him by the colonial government. The colonial state was essentially based on surveillance[52] and colonial officials such as Superintendents were given the dual responsibility of acquiring and implementing knowledge. Institutions such as asylums were part of this surveillance machinery. The maintenance of the lunatic asylum thus made it necessary for the Superintendent to study and observe people inside and outside the asylums.

A 'native' doctor resided on the premises and performed much of the medical and supervisory tasks. There is complete silence in the archives regarding the training and education of the 'native' doctor. However, he often had some education and, at times, also had medical training of some sort. Since the 1880s a Deputy Superintendent was appointed regularly in the asylums. He helped in the everyday functioning of the institution along with the Hospital Attendant, the Head Attendant, and the Matron. The Deputy Superintendents were usually of European origin, as were the Matrons. The Head Attendant, the other Hospital Attendants, as well as the subordinate staff were Indians. Every asylum had a few European patients who could only be taken care of by the white staff. The European staff was thus pertinent to maintaining the racial difference. The 'native' doctor was a vital link between the patient and the superior white authorities. He was familiar with the local practices, customs, and language. Ernst asserts that 'this system of dual management was intended to increase discipline and to establish social hierarchy within the asylum which was congruent with the reality of colonial rule'.[53]

[51] Waltraud Ernst, 'Institutions, People and Power: Lunatic Asylums in Bengal, c. 1800–1900', in *The Social History of Health and Medicine in Colonial India*, edited by Biswamoy Pati and Mark Harrison (London: Routledge, 2009), 139.

[52] For details, see C. A. Bayly, *Empire and Information: Intelligence Gathering and Social Communication in India, 1750–1870* (New Delhi: Cambridge University Press, 1999); Bernard S. Cohn, *Colonialism and Its Forms of Knowledge*, in *The Bernard Cohn Omnibus* (New Delhi: Oxford University Press, 2008).

[53] Waltraud Ernst, 'Idioms of Madness and Colonial Boundaries: The Case of the European and "Native" Mentally Ill in Early Nineteenth-Century British India', *Comparative Studies in Society and History*, vol. 39, no. 1 (1997): 160.

The asylum reports are replete with examples of assistance that the Indian subordinate staff rendered, and the obstacles they placed in everyday working of the asylum. At the end of each asylum report, the Superintendent gave a detailed description of the functioning of the staff. He applauded the efficiency of the staff at times and, at other times, complained about the unavailability of efficient subordinate staff. James H. Mills had examined the day-to-day workings of the lunatic asylums in India. These asylums were managed by the Indian subordinate staff. He argues that 'the Indian staff, who often had their own ideas about what should go on, actually determined condition and experiences. They at times frustrated and disrupted the management plans but, worked meticulously at others.'[54]

There were also constant complaints regarding the non-availability of good attendants. James Cleghorn, the Inspector General of Civil Hospitals, Punjab, wrote to R. E. Younghusband, the Junior Secretary to the Government of the Punjab, that 'the superintendents of both Asylums [Delhi and Lahore] complain of the indifferent class of men employed as warders. The rate of pay being much lower than that given in jails, renders it impossible to secure the services of efficient men.'[55] G. F. W. Ewens, the Superintendent of the Punjab asylum, stated in the Annual Report for the Year 1902:

> The inmates, as a whole, form a far more dangerous, noisy and trouble-some class and are infinitely more difficult to properly supervise, especially when it is remembered that the attendants obtainable here are of a very low order while they are also few in point of number. Rightly or wrongly, the fact remains that the duties of an attendant in the asylum are consid-ered as objectionable, and though the pay is relatively good, it is extremely difficult and rare to obtain men of good standard. No pensioned sepoy will undertake the work or stay at it more than a few days, except Mazbi Sikhs [i.e., Sikhs who have Dalit origins], and the more rational lunatics object to on the ground of caste. The increased pay in the higher grade attracts a certain number of reliable men, and those of long service often attain to a good practical knowledge of the peculiarities and modes of managing

---

54 Mills, *Madness, Cannabis and Colonialism*, 158–159.

55 The Annual Report of the Lunatic Asylums of the Punjab for the Year 1893, NAI.

individual patients. Still the general number leave much to be desired. The strictest and most careful supervision is exercised to prevent any harshness and abuse of power, and such cases are severely dealt with. As a result one can confidently assert that very few instances arise. The female attendants obtainable are of very low order, and compare very unfavourably with the male, and for this no remedy seems at present forthcoming.[56]

Moreover, notions of caste were seen as obstacles to the appointment of attendants and nurses. For instance, the Mazhbi Sikhs were members of lower castes who had embraced the Sikh faith. Attendants belonging to lower castes were considered problematic due to their untouchable status in Indian society. The lunatics often refused to eat or drink from their hands. Even their presence was at times objected to.[57] In this rigid milieu, the staff belonging to the lower castes lived on the margins because of the hatred that they had to face from the patients and personnel. More recent research on the Bombay asylum highlights that 'most of the subordinate staff in the Bombay's asylum came from *Mahar* and *Madrasi* communities … While pay, promotions and accommodation were good incentives for the subordinate staff, service in the asylum gave them a means to break free from economic and psychological subservience to existing village structures.'[58] The economic

---

[56] The Annual Report of the Lunatic Asylum of the Punjab for the Year 1902, National Medical Library.

[57] There exists a number of works on the status of the lower castes in colonial and postcolonial India. Some of these works have argued that the colonial state failed to emancipate the lower castes. The colonial education system further entrenched the caste rigidities as education in the colonial period was only available to the high castes. The lower castes thus failed to rise in the compartmentalized hierarchical structures and were forced to do menial jobs. For further reference, see Dilip Menon, *Caste, Nationalism and Communism in Malabar* (Cambridge: Cambridge, 1994); Vijay Prasad, *Untouchable Freedom: A Social History of a Dalit Community* (New Delhi, Oxford University Press, 2000); Mark Jurgensmeyer, *Religion as Social Vision: The Movement against Untouchability in Twentieth Century Punjab* (Berkeley: University of California Press, 1982); Vidhya Raveendranathan, 'Constructing the Scavenger: Caste and Labour in Colonial South India, 1860–1940', unpublished MPhil dissertation, Department of History, University of Delhi, 2011.

[58] Pinto, 'Shackled Bodies, Unchained Minds', 76–7.

and social status gained by working for the colonial bureaucracy was considered a serious incentive that provided a push to the lower castes and classes to work in rather unpopular institutions such as the 'mad-houses' in colonial India.

Some significant attempts were nevertheless made to raise the salary of these attendants. However, the increase was minimal. T. E. L. Bate, the Inspector General of Civil Hospitals, Punjab, noted in the Triennial Report of the Years 1906–8:

> It is unfortunate that the large enhancement of the scale of wages of the attendants, sanctioned by Government in 1907, has been nullified by the great increase that has taken place in the market rate of labour during the past few years. The duties the keepers have to perform are extremely distasteful, and it is very doubtful whether any reasonable remuneration would induce men of a suitable type to take the service; if men of the proper stamp are to be had at any price in this country.[59]

Attempts were again made in 1916 to raise the salaries of the attendants. C. Mactaggar, the Inspector General of Civil Hospital, stated in the Triennial Report for the Lunatic Asylum in the United Provinces (1915, 1916, and 1917),

> To meet the difficulty experienced in securing suitable candidates as female warders, government revised the scale of pay of these employees with effect from the 1st March, 1916. In September of the same year it was ruled that the entire service of head warders, including the service rendered by them as warders, should be treated as superior for purposes of pension.[60]

Superintendents and visiting officers were sympathetic to the conditions of the attendants. These concerns often arose due to the unpopularity and scarcity of people interested in working in the asylums.

Female attendants were more difficult to find than males. Given the socio-economic conditions and entrenched patriarchical norms, there

---

[59] The Triennial Report on the Lunatic Asylum in the Punjab for the Years 1906, 1907, and 1908, National Medical Library.

[60] The Triennial Report on the Lunatic Asylums in the United Provinces for the Years 1916, 1917, and 1918 NAI.

would have been very few women who would have been willing to work in mental institutions. The work in these institutions was regarded as too dangerous and unpleasant. Franciscan nuns belonging to a Catholic order were active in the Lahore asylum almost since the beginning of the twentieth century. They took control of the female section of the asylum. Year after year, the asylum reports commended their work. According to Ewens,

> The female insane is, however, fortunate in being entrusted to the care of four Franciscan nuns as matrons whose services are all the more appreciated as the only class of native woman to be obtained as an attendant is immeasurably inferior even to those among the men and who are wanting in even the rudiments of intelligence or energy.[61]

This sort of comparison was demeaning and racial in nature. The work of the Franciscan nuns in the asylum was much admired by the Lieutenant Governor of the Punjab and the Viceroy of India. Fr Leo, O.M. Cap., in an article entitled 'The Franciscan Sisters at the Lunatic Asylum' while writing about his experience stated:

> On his visit to the Asylum in April 1906, Sir Charles Rivaz, Lt. Governor of the Punjab, was struck with astonishment at the happy results of the work of the sisters and to show his deep appreciation, he wrote these flattering remarks in the Visitor's Book of the Asylum: 'The Female Asylum is generally a pleasing contrast to the Male Asylum, partly because there is sufficient accommodation, but mainly because it has the good fortune to be under the management of four Roman Catholic sisters, who live in the Asylum and give up their whole time to it. The moral influence which these ladies have evidently acquired over the patients by their cheerful demeanour, and kindly and paternal treatment of them, is very remarkable, and the excellent work they are doing under what are necessarily very trying circumstances cannot be overestimated.' This need of praise, coming from a Protestant official, speaks volumes for the work of our Sisters.[62]

---

[61] The Triennial Report on the Lunatic Asylum in the Punjab for the Years 1906, 1907, and 1908, National Medical Library.

[62] Fr Leo, O. M. Cap., *Missionary Apostolate in the Punjab* (Mangalore: Codialbail Press, 1910), 102–3. (I owe this particular reference to Dr Radha Kapuria.)

In 1910, the Franciscan nuns were awarded for their active philan-thropic work in the asylum. R. Humphreys, the Revenue Secretary of the Government, Punjab, noted in the Annual Report for the Lunatic Asylum for the Year 1910 that the Franciscan sisters were publicly pre-sented with the badge of Kaisar-i-Hind by the Viceroy.[63] However, by the 1930s their work began to be regarded as 'unprofessional'. C. J. Lodge Patch, the Superintendent of the Punjab Mental Hospital, observed in the Triennial Reports for the Years 1930–2:

> For 30 years the Mental Hospital for Women has been supervised by Franciscan Nuns. Apart from the fact that these ladies had had practi-cally no training in modern hospital methods, many administrative difficulties were experienced ... the Government paid them larger sala-ries than most trained nursing sisters. The greatest praise is due to some of these Franciscan Nuns, particularly the late Mother Simon, Mother Veronica and Sister Eleanore. But the decision of Government to replace them by a staff of five trained hospital nursing sisters will undoubtedly increase efficiency.[64]

In 1885 steps for the training of nurses and attendants in England were initiated. The Medico-Psychological Association also published a *Handbook for the Instruction of Attendants on the Insane* also known as *The Red Book* to disseminate information on the subject.[65] From 1891 onwards, the nurses and attendants associated with mental health were given practical training and had to pass an examination.[66] These measures notwithstanding, Indian personnel did not receive proper training. The attendants working in Indian asylums usually belonged to the lower strata of society and had very little or no education.

[63] The Annual Report on the Lunatic Asylum in the Punjab for the Year 1910, National Medical Library.

[64] The Triennial Report of the Punjab Mental Hospital for the Years 1930, 1931, and 1932, National Medical Library.

[65] See C. Chatterton, '"Caught in the Middle"? Mental Nurse Training in England 1919–51', *Journal of Psychiatric and Mental Health Nursing*, vol. 11, no. 1 (2004): 31.

[66] See Henry Rollin, 'Psychiatry in Britain One Hundred Years Ago', *The British Journal of Psychiatry*, vol. 183, no. 10 (2003): 295.

An attempt was made to introduce training for nurses of mental asylums when in 1932 training at St Andrew's Hospital in Northampton and its certificate obtained official recognition in India.[67] Therefore, professionalization of Indian attendants did not occur in a proper manner.

The Indian subordinate staff were sometimes appreciated for their contribution but were rarely rewarded. It would not be wrong to state that the asylum subordinate staff faced discrimination, violence, and instability as far as their jobs were concerned. They were frequently dismissed in instances where patients escaped or committed suicide. A number of examples can be cited to show how the attendants were fined, punished, or dismissed. C. A. Sprawson, the Inspector General of Civil Hospitals pointed out in the Triennial Report for the Mental Hospitals of the United Provinces for the Years 1927, 1928, and 1929, 'The number of escapes from the Agra Mental Hospital must be attributed partly to shortness of staff and partly to slackness and corruption on the part of some attendants. In the latter cases disciplinary action was taken.'[68] F. Fleming, the Superintendent of the Punjab Lunatic Asylum mentioned in the Triennial Report of 1915, 1916, and 1917,

> In 1910 and 1917 there were 3 and 2 escapes, respectively. Of these 2 were soon returned to the asylum. These escapes usually occur from the garden gangs and in all cases are due to the absolute carelessness of the attendants in charge, who show no sense of responsibility. In all cases the attendants culpable has been severely punished. The system of criminally prosecuting the attendants at fault in certain cases has proved efficacious though it cannot be very widely adopted at the present time owing to the difficulty of obtaining labour of any description.[69]

[67] Enquiry as to the Recognition in India of the Certificate in Mental Nursing by the Royal Medico-Psychological Association, St Andrew Hospital, Northampton, Home/Jails, File No. 124, 1932, NAI.

[68] The Triennial Report for the Mental Hospitals for the United Provinces for the Year 1927, 1928, and 1929, NAI.

[69] The Triennial Report on the Lunatic Asylum of the Punjab for the Years 1915, 1916, and 1917, National Medical Library.

Being located on the lowest rung of the hierarchy, attendants were subject to double violence. At one level they had to cope with constant humiliation by the white authorities and at another level they were subjected to violence at the hands of the insane. Overcrowding and lack of staff were common phenomena. Lack of training and lack of status, along with discriminatory wages marred the efficiency of the Indian subordinate staff. Shula Marks, who has studied the status and condition of mental nurses in South Africa during the first half of the twentieth century, notes in the context that 'the desperate overcrowding of patients, and the paucity of staff, their "appalling" living conditions, lack of adequate training and lack of status meant that they were themselves under tremendous pressure'.[70]

Diagnosis and Categories

Historians of psychiatry concede the fact that segregation and incarceration of the insane is a modern phenomenon. Roy Porter has pointed out that 'more formal segregation began to emerge towards the end of the middle ages, often inspired by the Christian duty of charity'.[71] The Bethlehem or Bedlam was the earliest asylum that was established in London as early as 1247. It was founded under the auspices of the religious order of St Mary of Bethlehem.[72] However, it was not before the eighteenth century that organized efforts were made to develop a system for regulating lunacy. The diagnosis and categorization of madness in the modern period has also been a long drawn out process, which started with 'the rise of the asylum' as a special institution to incarcerate the 'mad'.

The mad were treated as vagrants in England before the Vagrancy Act of 1744. Vieda Skultans points out that 'the vagrancy act of

---

[70] Shula Marks, 'The Microphysics of Power: Mental Nursing in South Africa in the First Half of the Twentieth Century', in *Psychiatry and Empire*, edited by Sloan Mahone and Megan Vaughan (Basingstoke: Palgrave Macmillan 2007), 90.

[71] Roy Porter, *Madness: A Brief History* (Oxford: Oxford University Press, 2002), 90.

[72] Porter, Madness, 90.

1744 first made separate mention of lunatics.[73] Section 20 of the Act stated,

> It shall and may be lawful for any two or more Justices of the Peace where such lunatics and mad persons shall be found, by warrant under their hands and seals, directed to the constables, churchwardens and overseers of the poor of such Parish, Town or Place, to cause such persons to be apprehended and kept safely locked up in some secure place as such Justices shall appoint; and (if such Justices find it necessary) to be there chained.[74]

This measure gradually led to the management and the regulation of lunacy. In fact, the earliest attempts targeted what was then called 'trade in lunacy'. A number of private madhouses gave shelter to rich lunatics whose relatives regarded them as an embarrassment.[75] Since 1774 the private asylums were regulated by issuing legal licences in England.[76] Parliamentary Select Committees of 1805, 1815, and 1827 threw light on the plight of the criminal and the pauper insane. It was only from 1845 onwards that every county was required to have its own asylums. The Lunatics Act of 1845 also had mandatory provisions for pauper lunatics.[77]

British India had no vagrancy laws. Vagrancy laws meant provisions had to be made for the poor which was not feasible since poverty was not recognized as a problem in the colony. David Arnold remarks,

> Indians were deemed too numerous to receive systematic relief, and, anyways as the influential administrator and evangelical Charles Grant argued giving further weight to the naturalization of Indian poverty, they lived in a country where climate and customs have combined 'to keep

---

[73] Vieda Skultans, *English Madness: Ideas on Insanity, 1580–1890* (London: Routledge, 1979), 106.

[74] Skultans, *English Madness*, 106.

[75] For a discussion on private asylums in England, see William Parry-Jones, *The Trade in Lunacy: A Study of Private Madhouses in England in the Eighteenth and Nineteenth Centuries* (London: Routledge & Kegan Paul, 1972).

[76] In 1774, the Act for Regulating Private Madhouses was passed in England.

[77] Skultans, *English Madness*, 98.

down the standards of wants among the Indian poor. The tropical climate minimizes the need for food and artificial warmth and so simplifies the mere act of living.[78]

Vagrancy, however, was considered to be a greater threat in the colonies. The colonial state, thus, devised an array of laws to deal with vagrant and nomadic ways of life. Darwin's discoveries added a hue of criminality to vagrancy.[79] This had severe repercussions in the colonies where a whole set of communities and tribes were labelled as criminals. Tim Lloyd has closely looked at the 'Anti-Thugee Campaign' (1829–41). In the colonial period, 'thugs' were considered to be professional criminals who looted and killed innocent people and travellers. He contends that in the colonial period, 'thugee' as a category was expounded and exploited by the colonial state which was attempting to establish its political sovereignty in the early years of the Company Raj. Llyod argues,

> The historiographical claim here is that 'colonial sovereignty' names a type of power that British administrators demanded, and instituted, for the control of certain individuals whose actions transgressed the threshold of their modes of comprehension and categorization. 'Thug' was the name given to a figure located beyond the pale of 'civil' society, and held to be a member of a community of irreclaimable predators upon it, who could not be socialized into conventional law.[80]

Kim Wagner noted that 'the men involved [in Thuggee] were part of the military labour market, sometimes joining larger armies and sometimes serving petty zemindars, and when faced by demobilization they had to find other ways of gaining a livelihood. In other words: Thuggee was

---

[78] David Arnold, 'Vagrant India: Famine, Poverty and Welfare under Colonial Rule', in *Cast Out: Vagrancy and Homelessness in Global and Historical Perspective*, edited by A. L. Beier and Paul Ocobock (Ohio: Ohio University Press, 2008), 121.

[79] For further details, see Meena Radhakrishna, 'Of Apes and Ancestors: Evolutionary Science and Colonial Ethnography', *The Indian Historical Review*, vol. 33, no. 1 (2006): 1–23.

[80] Tom Lloyd, 'Thuggee, Marginality and the State Effect in Colonial India, circa 1770–1840', *Indian Economic and Social History Review*, vol. 45, no. 2 (2008): 233.

the continuation of a predatory lifestyle.'[81] Therefore, the suppression of 'thuggee' was actually destruction of these itinerant ways of life. These efforts continued throughout the nineteenth century during which a number of attempts were made to control those communities and individuals who were considered irascible and dangerous. The Criminal Tribes Act of 1871 was one such prominent mechanism. Meena Radhakrishna points out that 'the ostensible purpose of the Criminal Tribes Act of 1871 had been to suppress "hereditary criminal" sections of Indian society.'[82] She further comments that the Criminal Tribes Act 'arose out of policies of political control rather than social concern for escalating crime.'[83]

There were, however, groups that could not be bought under the purview of the law. It would thus not be far-fetched to argue that policies pertaining to lunacy attempted to bring these 'irascible' individuals and groups under the political control of the state. 'Madness' as a term encompassed various forms of deviancies ranging from vagrancy to spirit drinking to hemp drug use. The so-called delinquents were considered dangerous and thus were shut away in the asylums. An analysis of these groups would further allow us to unravel the nature of psychiatry. Mills has used the case notes of the Lucknow asylum to throw light on the kind of people who were incarcerated. He shows through these case notes that the wanderers were considered to be a menace and threat:

> Act XXXVI of 1858 ... gave the colonial authorities the power to detain all those individuals that they considered to be 'wandering' and 'lurking' in their districts. These legislative provisions dealing with individuals should be seen alongside legalisation like the Criminal Tribes Act of 1871 ... this act was aimed at providing a legal framework within which the colonial state could prevent the movement of whole groups of Indians. The nomadic lifestyle of the communities identified in these acts were rendered illegal by the colonial state and systems were established to manage and prevent those lifestyles. Provisions included having suspect

---

[81] Kim Wagner, 'The Deconstructed Stranglers: A Reassessment of Thuggee', *Modern Asian Studies*, vol. 38, no. 4 (2004): 963.

[82] Radhakrishna, *Dishonoured by History*, 2.

[83] Radhakrishna, *Dishonoured by History*, 4.

tribes register themselves in fixed places and necessitated the possession of a license before travelling.[84]

These categories included spirit users, hemp and opium users, and mendicants (yogis, faqirs, *qalandars*, and *sadhus*). These were people who were generally very poor. Economic changes had left many of them unemployed. Poor laws and pauper lunacy laws were based on the basic assumption of differentiating individuals on the basis of their ability to work. Since colonial India did not have workhouses in the European sense, lunatic asylums became the abode of these people. Madness and delinquency were, thus, coterminous in colonial India.

The first category of such delinquents was that of the hemp users. From the 1850s onwards hemp started getting linked to insanity. Consumption of hemp was linked to crime, immorality, and insanity. The drug came under close scrutiny when the colonial state set up the IHDC in 1893 (see discussion on the IHDC in Chapter 1). It aimed to probe the moral, social, economic, and mental effects of the use of hemp. The IHDC concluded that 'there was no trustworthy basis for a satisfactory and reasonably accurate opinion on the connection between hemp drugs and insanity in the asylum statistics appended to the annual report'.[85] It also declared hemp to be a part of the Indian social and cultural milieus.

The IHDC's denial of links between hemp, immorality, crime, and insanity was to a great extent determined by the fact that hemp generated a significant amount of revenue which the state could not easily forgo. Under the circumstances, a better policy was to incarcerate hemp users in asylums. The supposed association between hemp and insanity diminished but the link never vanished. Jal Edulji Dhunjibhoy, the Superintendent of Indian Mental Hospital, Kanke, Ranchi, wrote an article on hemp insanity in 1930.[86] He described in detail the

[84] Mills, *Madness, Cannabis and Colonialism*, 72.

[85] Report of the Indian Hemp Drugs Commission 1893–1894, vol. I (Simla: Government Central Printing Office, 1894), 237.

[86] Jal Edulji Dhunjibhoy, 'A Brief Résumé of the Types of Insanity Commonly Met with in the Country India, with a Full Description of "Indian Hemp Insanity" Peculiar to the Country', *Journal of Mental Sciences*, vol. 76 (1930).

preparation method of ganja, *charas*, and *bhang* and discussed the ways in which they were consumed. According to him there were three types of hemp insanity:'(1) Acute mania, (2) chronic mania, and (3) dementia. The difference between these types is only a question of degree'.[87] He also underlined the supposed connection between crime and insanity. Dhunjibhoy claimed that 'excessive or prolonged use of hemp drugs degrades the mind and character of the consumer and predisposes him to commit crime. Thus hemp is one of the most effectual means of increasing the criminal classes in India. It is also largely consumed by bad characters to fortify themselves for crime'.[88] He had internalized colonial notions of a link between hemp insanity and crime which was then termed as 'hemp psychosis'.

Even though opium was not considered to be as harmful as hemp, it was nevertheless seen as one of the causes of insanity. The Civil Surgeon of the Dacca asylum wrote that 'there is always a small proportion of the inmate whose mental condition has been ruined by opium smoking or eating it ... opium-eating is general among the Mahommedans of this district after middle age'.[89] Ewens noted that 'alcohol is a very important cause, either directly or as a toxin indirectly by its leading to want and worry, and its influence in causing degenerate, vicious and idiotic children is indubitable'.[90] Dhunjibhoy regarded toxic substances as one of the major reasons for insanity:

(a) In this group hemp drug tops the list. (b) Alcohol is second. Alcohol is largely consumed in those parts of India where the hemp drug is difficult

[87] Dhunjibhoy, 'A Brief Résumé of the Types of Insanity', 232.

[88] Dhunjibhoy, 'A Brief Résumé of the Types of Insanity', 234.

[89] Sir James Clark's Enquiry as to the Care and the Treatment of Lunatics, Home Dept./Public Branch, File No. 22–23, 19 December 1868, NAI.

[90] G. F. W. Ewens, *Insanity in India: Its Symptoms and Diagnosis: With Reference to the Relation of Crime and Insanity* (Calcutta: Thacker, Spink & Co., 1908, reprinted in Memphis by General Books, 2009), 21. During the latter half of the nineteenth century, a clear link between alcohol and degeneration was forged in Europe. The play between alcoholism, degeneration, and madness can be seen in Emile Zola's novel *L'Assommoir* (1877). Alcohol was not linked to insanity in the Indian context, whereas hemp was regarded as one of the primary cause of insanity in the Indian lunatic asylums.

to obtain or is unknown. The types of alcoholic psychosis are the same as one seen in the West. The consumption of opium and cocaine is by no means less in India than elsewhere, yet the mental disorders due to over indulgence in these drugs are not often seen; in fact, they are very rare. (c) Acute confusional insanity is also not uncommon in India, and in a good many cases the principal aetiological factors are starvation and physical exhaustion. Such cases make a speedy recovery with rest and a good nourishing diet.[91]

The records of the period also reflect the worry of the Europeans concerning the overt sexuality of 'natives'. Excessive sexual intercourse and masturbation were often linked to insanity and the degenerate civilization of India.

A closer look at the changing classification and treatment would help us in understanding the changing nature of psychiatry in the colonies. During the first half of the nineteenth century the basic categories of insanity were mania (acute or chronic) and melancholia (acute or chronic). Epilepsy and idiocy were seen as distinct from other forms of insanity. Certain forms of insanity were regarded to be commonly found in India whereas the absence of others was considered to be peculiar. Ernst notes that 'this contention was supported by ideas on the impact of warm climates on the body and mind and beliefs in racial difference'.[92] Dr Scriven, Superintendent of the Lahore asylum, pointed out in the Annual Report of 1871:

> The classification of the forms of madness as manifested in natives is, in my opinion susceptible of a more simple arrangement ... in which we have acute and chronic mania, and also acute and chronic dementia. Instead of these four heads, I would make two great forms of mental derangement, one characterized by visible excitement, the other by depression. Melancholia, when the mind is engrossed in some painful sentiment, with perhaps propensity to suicide or homicidal impulse, may complicate almost every form of derangement of mind, but it is always dependent on delusion expressed or not, and, therefore, is correctly made a separate

---

[91] Dhunjibhoy, 'A Brief Résumé of the Types of Insanity', 256.

[92] Waltraud Ernst, *Colonialism and Transnational Psychiatry: The Development of an Indian Mental Hospital in British India, c. 1925–1940* (London: Anthem Press, 2013), 137.

disorder. Females are more subject to melancholia than males. I think [general paralysis of insane], which one so often sees and hears of in the Lunatic Asylums at home, is not common out here, in fact, in my little experience in India I think it is very rare. Idiocy of course comes under a separate heading. Epileptic mania is very common and has been placed under chronic mania.[93]

There existed a popular notion that insanity was induced by the stress of 'civilization'. 'Nomads' and 'uncivilized races' were supposedly closer to nature and thus insanity was not that widely prevalent among them. A simple arrangement of categories was thus considered enough in the case of colonies. Nonetheless, it was held that insanity in India was often 'self-induced' (because of the use of hemp and other kinds of narcotic addictions) and hence more easily treatable than in civilized societies.[94]

The belief that madness and mental weakness were hereditary traits gained ground in Europe in the period. Rafael Huertas has pointed out:

At the beginning of the nineteenth century important changes occurred in biological sciences. European and American society reacted to the publication of *On the Origin of Species* as if they feared the novelties evolutionism could bring. Anthropological racism, medical somaticism, persecution of the abnormal or the unusual, and so forth, were some of the major contributions of positivist science ... in this context, doctors examined criminals and the mentally ill in an attempt to provide scientific and even philosophical support for the demands of fin de siècle bourgeois society.[95]

Benedict Augustin Morel (1809–1873), Cesare Lombroso, (1835–1909), and Henry Maudsley (1835–1918) popularized the notion that madness was the result of degeneration. Richard D. Walter has pointed

[93] The Annual Report of the Lunatic Asylums of the Punjab for the Year 1871, NAI.

[94] Proposal for the construction for the Lunatic Asylum at Agra, Home Dept./Public Branch, File No. 26 to 30, 20 October 1862, NAI.

[95] Rafael Huertas and C. M. Winston, 'Madness and Degeneration, I: From "Fallen Angel" to Mentally Ill', *History of Psychiatry*, vol. 3, no. 4 (1992): 391–2.

out that for Morel, degeneration was 'a progressive, or really retrogressive, process in which the influence of diet, toxins, climate, disease, and moral depravities of one generation induced a high proportion of neurotics, criminals, and paupers in the next generation.'[96] People such as Maudsley criticized the asylum system. He believed that the numbers of insane were increasing but the asylums could not treat insanity. Maudsley believed that insanity was inherited and was the result of degeneration. Lombroso tried to establish links between crime, insanity, and physical features. By studying physical features such as jaws, nasal index, and cheek bones, Lombroso claimed to have figured out degenerates who had atavistic tendencies.

Ideas of degeneration and hereditarianism were part of broader racial understanding. Certain 'races' were considered to be more prone to crime and insanity than others. The identification of supposed racial mental characteristics with mental illnesses was the product of such notions. Ewens stated in his 1905 monograph that

> the ... heredity [hereditary result] direct or indirect of disease, injury, sunstroke, abuse of alcoholic or other intoxicants, bad livings, unhealthy climatic and social environment, [is that] children are born with a vitiated degenerated constitution, [which is] more and more evident as these morbid influences have been repeated in former generations and the only possible diminution by the atavism to some more healthy predecessor.[97]

Hereditary insanity as a category had by now emerged in asylum records. A. W. Overbeck-Wright wrote in 1920 that 'a *tainted heredity* figure[s] very prominently among etiological factors. If we include cases with a tainted family history along with those with a personal history or signs of degeneracy, then some 440 of the 2,346 admissions are afflicted from this cause.'[98] Racial profiling occurred at several levels during this period. The Ethnographic Survey of India had entered a vigorous phase

---

[96] Richard D. Walter, 'What Became of the Degenerate? A Brief History of a Concept', *Journal of the History of Medicine*, vol. 11, no. 4 (1956): 423.

[97] Ewens, *Insanity in India*, 170.

[98] Alexander William Overbeck-Wright, *Lunacy in India* (London: Bailliere, Tindall and Cox, 1921), 7.

from 1901 onwards, that is, with the appointment of H. H. Risley as its Director. W. W. Hunter had once remarked that India was a 'great museum of races in which one can study man from his lowest to highest stages of culture'.[99] The diverse social groups of India were measured on the evolutionary scale of civilization. This led to the hierarchization of their physical and mental characteristics. Some communities and castes were regarded as martial and intelligent and thus superior, while others were considered weak and feeble-minded and therefore inferior. For example, once the notions about 'martial races' became prevalent, the Punjabis were regarded as 'brave' and 'manly'. However, in the asylum their manliness was understood in terms of a propensity towards violence. H. W. V. Cox, the Superintendent of the Punjab Lunatic Asylum asserted that 'the characteristic features of the Punjabi insane are violence and destructiveness, and they are even more pronounced in the Pathan, of whom there are a very large number'.[100] Excuses for dysfunctional workings of the asylum were also offered in racial terms. Patch, the Superintendent of Punjab Mental Hospital wrote, 'Indeed, the harmless, non-criminal garden worker is infinitely less dangerous than a large proportion of the insane who are still in their own towns and villages'.[101] Indians were largely regarded as insane whether inside or outside the asylums. This racial difference along with financial constraints were cited as a justification for a number of inadequacies in the psychiatric infrastructure.

Insanity was believed to be caused by moral and physical factors. Moral causes included worry, grief, loss of property, and even religion in the Indian context. Madness caused due to emotional factors was loosely known as moral insanity. Physical factors ranged from the use of hemp to spirit drinking and from heredity to epilepsy. The distinctions were often arbitrary. In the colonial context, degeneration blurred the

[99] W. W. Hunter, *The Indian Empire: Its History, People and Products* (London: Trubner and Co, 1882), 58, cited in Radhakrishna, 'Of Apes and Ancestors': 8.

[100] The Triennial Report on the Lunatic Asylum in the Punjab for the Years 1915, 1916, and 1917, National Medical Library.

[101] The Triennial Report on the Mental Hospital in the Punjab for the Years 1930, 1931, and 1932, National Medical Library.

difference between moral and physical causes. Diagnosis of insanity and attribution of a cause for it had become vague. Sally Swartz points out,

> Mental illness, a form of degeneration, and symbolizing the confrontation between civilization and savagery, through the person of the deranged lunatic, became an arena within which colonial authorities formulated their response to otherness ... thus degeneracy theory, and the evolutionary ideology it carried, explained the cause and perceived spread of mental illness and also justified domination of one group by another.[102]

By the first decade of the twentieth century, new categories were invented and older ones were widened. This reflected changes occurring in the field in Western Europe. E. L. Ward, Superintendent in Charge of the Punjab Lunatic Asylum, observed in the Triennial Report on the Lunatic Asylum of the Punjab for the Years 1912, 1913, and 1914:

> Dementia Praecox shows an increasing number. Idiopathic Mania and Melancholia (the German Mania Depressive) which was formerly so rare out here exhibits a gradually increasing number and is found chiefly amongst the more literate class of patients, a feature which should not be lost sight of as years go on, an indication of an increase in the growing education of the general population.[103]

The German manic depression and dementia praecox would later be known in the twentieth century as bipolar disorder and schizophrenia respectively. The idea that the advancement of civilization is linked to an increase in diseases was crucial as it was believed that some of these diseases were more common among the civilized and literate classes. Numerous developments were taking place in Europe, especially in Germany, at this time. Some of the important figures who changed the face of psychiatry emerged during this period. Franz Joseph Gall and J. C. Spurheim were anatomists who maintained that insanity could be understood by comprehending the overall topography ('hills and valleys')

---

[102] Sally Swartz, 'Colonizing the Insane: Causes of Insanity in the Cape', *History of the Human Sciences*, vol. 8, no. 4 (1995): 39–40.

[103] The Triennial Report on the Lunatic Asylum of the Punjab for the Years 1912, 1913, and 1914, National Medical Library.

of the brain.[104] Richard von Krafft-Ebing brought a number of sexual conditions under the yoke of psychiatry. These conditions ranged from homosexuality to transvestism and from bestiality to exhibitionism. Emil Kraepelin developed the concept of dementia praecox that later on was known as schizophrenia. Eugen Bleuler was a Swiss psychiatrist who for the first time used the term 'schizophrenia'. Among the famous German psychiatrists a name that should be mentioned is of course that of Sigmund Freud whose notions of the conscious and the unconscious had a much deeper influence on the practice of curing and dealing with insanity. These changes should be understood against the backdrop of Social Darwinism and the notion of degeneration that shaped developments in psychiatry.

Treatment and Medicines

Enlightenment rationality had given rise to confidence in dealing with insanity. Pinel's act of freeing the insane from shackles reflected this enthusiasm and assurance of triumph over irrationality. As stated before, moral management was widely accepted as a method of managing insanity in the nineteenth century. The basic principles of moral management were observation and control. This control would enable lunatics to develop their willpower and allow them to differentiate between right and wrong. Moral management was popular in Indian asylums. The Superintendents of asylums were well-acquainted with the moral management system. In the words of Dr Penny, the Superintendent of the Delhi asylum:

> I believe that scrupulous cleanliness, liberal diet, affording them means of recreation or occupation, and attention to the function of body are the foundation of the medical treatment and moral management of lunatics. ... Good feeding, great kindness and indulgence of every harmless kind, strict cleanliness, tobacco and carefully watching all the functions of body contribute towards the relief of these most unhappy sufferers.[105]

[104] Porter, *Madness*, 143.

[105] The Annual Report of the Lunatic Asylums of the Punjab for the Year 1871, NAI.

Nevertheless, the evidence suggests that throughout the nineteenth century restraint in one form or another was resorted to. The Civil Surgeon of the Lucknow asylum pointed out that 'the only restraint employed is the straitjacket and this is only used in the most extreme cases, and then for a very short time. This occasion does not happen once a month [*sic*]. There are three jackets in the store room'.[106] The Superintendent in Charge of the Moydnapore asylum exclaimed that 'handcuffs are now and then resorted to. None is kept in the asylum, but when required, have been borrowed from the jail, which is near at hand'.[107] In England blood-letting was regarded as controversial since Philippe Pinel had discarded the practice. The Superintendent in Charge of the Patna asylum stated, 'I frequently resort to topical depletion, applying, as needs be, three to twelve leeches to each temple'.[108]

Dr Wise of the Dacca asylum pointed out that 'confinement in a solitary cell for a few hours, curtailing the daily allowance of tobacco, or prohibiting their attendance to the nautches, are found to be sufficient punishments for the mischievous and unmanageable patients'.[109] Every asylum had several solitary cells to sequester the refractory inmates (see Figure 2.3). Sometimes hot and cold baths were given to cure insanity. Dr Fairweather of the Delhi asylum wrote in 1875, 'Little treatment of a medical kind has been attempted except in cases of great excitement, when the warm bath with cold douche to the head has been found useful, or occasionally a dose of chloral hydrat, or a blister to the back of head'.[110] Blisters were commonly used in India to calm down the difficult patients. Sedatives such as hydrocyanic acid were believed to be beneficial in calming excitable patients. The Superintendent in Charge at the Bareilly asylum remarked that

---

[106] Sir James Clark's Enquiry as to the Care and the Treatment of Lunatics, Home Dept./Public Branch, File No. 22–23, 19 December 1868, NAI.

[107] Sir James Clark's Enquiry as to the Care and the Treatment of Lunatics, Home Dept./Public Branch, File No. 22–23, 19 December 1868, NAI.

[108] Sir James Clark's Enquiry as to the Care and the Treatment of Lunatics, Home Dept./Public Branch, File No. 22–23, 19 December 1868, NAI.

[109] Sir James Clark's Enquiry as to the Care and the Treatment of Lunatics, Home Dept./Public Branch, File No. 22–23, 19 December 1868, NAI.

[110] The Annual Report of the Lunatic Asylums of the Punjab for the Year 1875, NAI.

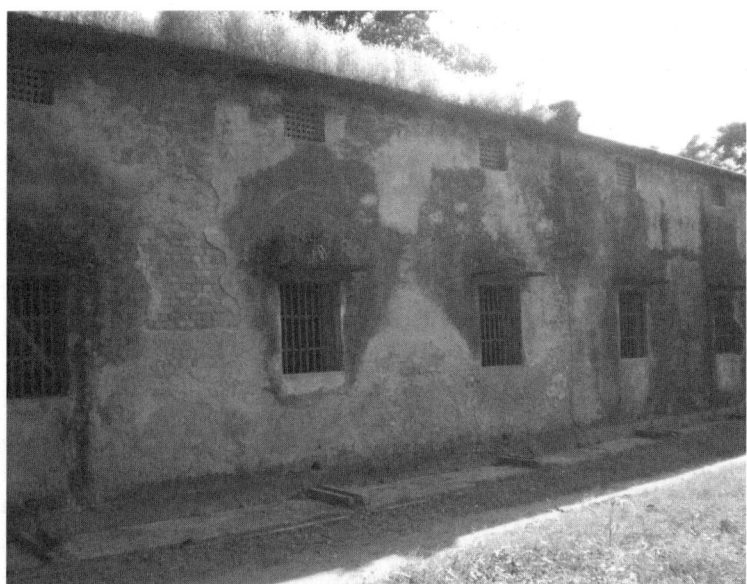

Figure 2.3   Ten solitary cells also known as Dus Kothi at the Bareilly Mental Hospital, photographed in 2012
Source: Author.

'the bromide of potassium has been found to be a valuable remedy in cases of insanity, accompanied by sleeplessness'.[111] Liberal diet, light labour, and amusement were considered imperative for the treatment of the insane. However, as we shall see in the next chapter, neither was the diet 'liberal' and nor was labour 'light'. Colonial psychiatry, in sum, had little to offer in the nineteenth century as far as the treatment of the insane was concerned.

By the end of the century, pessimism related to the cure rates of insanity had heightened. The asylums in the West were filled with 'incurables' as the number of 'cured' patients had dropped significantly. An answer to these problems was found in the larger philosophy of degeneration. Moral therapy came to be regarded as redundant as psychiatry

---

[111] Sir James Clark's Enquiry as to the Care and the Treatment of Lunatics, Home Dept./Public Branch, File No. 22–23, 19 December 1868, NAI.

took a biological turn. Edward Shorter has suggested the following in the context:

> In the first half of the twentieth century, psychiatry was caught in a dilemma. On the one hand, psychiatrists could warehouse their patients in vast bins in the hope that they might recover spontaneously. On the other, they had psychoanalysis, a therapy suitable for need of wealthy people desiring self-insight, but not for real psychiatric illness. Caught between these unappealing choices, psychiatrists sought alternatives. Some of these alternatives proved to be dead ends and were discarded; others became the basis of a new vision of psychotherapy; still others laid the groundwork for the revolution in drug therapy that would take place after WWII.[112]

Shorter's view belongs to the tradition of historians who view psychiatry's trajectory in triumphalist terms. Many therapies were experimented with in this period. Quite a few of these therapies were abandoned while others laid the basis of what is known today as 'modern' psychiatry.

In the early decades of the twentieth century, a number of fever, coma, and shock therapies were developed for dealing with insanity. A Viennese psychiatrist, Julius Wagner-Jauregg, discovered the cure of neurosyphilis in 1917. He inoculated a patient with malaria and administrated quinine and after some period of time, astonishingly, the patient's sphyilitic fits came to an end. Shorter remarks that the 'Wagner-Jauregg's fever "cure" (it did not cure but it did restore an almost normal life to patients who otherwise would have died demented) broke the therapeutic nihilism that dominated psychiatry in previous generations.'[113] In 1929, Knud Schroeder in Denmark developed the sulfosin therapy. The suspension of sulphur was used to induce fever of high grade and it was believed that it could treat various types of insanity. Ernst has observed that 'as early as in the year 1930, J. E. Dhunjibhoy, the superintendent of the Indian Mental Hospital at Ranchi used "Schroeder's formula" (of a 1% solution or suspension of sulphur in olive oil) and applied it to patients he had diagnosed with a range of

---

[112] Edward Shorter, *A History of Psychiatry: From the Era of the Asylum to the Age of Prozac* (New York: John Wiley & Sons, 1997), 190.

[113] Shorter, *A History of Psychiatry*, 194.

mental disorders, such as manic-depressive psychosis, dementia prae-cox and epilepsy.[114] It was only in the second half of the 1930s that sulphosin therapy, cardizol injections, and insulin therapies were intro-duced in the United Provinces and the Punjab asylums.[115] The Punjab Mental Hospital Report stated that 'in 1938 special forms of treatment by Cardiazol and Insulin were introduced and very promising results were obtained. Out of the 94 patients treated, 27 were "cured" and 31 "improved". Owing to the shortage of funds it was not possible to try the experiment on a large scale.[116] Hydrotherapy was also employed in the mental hospitals of the United Provinces.[117]

Manfred Sakel had introduced insulin shock therapy in 1933. Sakel had used doses of insulin to treat addicts and later on used larger quantities of it to induce coma and convulsions in order to treat schizophrenic patients. His experiments were soon adopted by other psychiatrists. In 1934 Ladislaus von Meduna induced fits in a schizophrenic patient with the help of pentamethylenetetrazol, a car-diac stimulant also known as Cardiazol or Metrazol. Niall McCrae has pointed out that 'results from Meduna's (1935) first 26 patients showed that 10 had completely recovered.[118] These methods soon became widespread and were practised all over the world. These were also adopted in India but their uses were restricted due to the high cost of these drugs. Ernst argues that in the context of Ranchi, 'it was a higher cost of particular treatments rather than lack of interest or knowledge that made it impossible for Dhunjibhoy to pioneer some of

---

[114] Waltraud Ernst, 'Practising "Colonial" or "Modern" Psychiatry in British India? Treatments at the Indian Mental Hospital at Ranchi, 1925–1940', in *Transnational Psychiatries: Social and Cultural Histories of Psychiatry in Comparative Perspective c. 1800–2000*, edited by Waltraud Ernst and Thomas Mueller (Newcastle: Cambridge Scholars Publishing), 92.

[115] The Triennial Report on Mental Hospitals in the United Provinces for the Years 1936, 1937, and 1938, NAI.

[116] The Annual Report on the Mental Hospital in the Punjab for the Year 1938, National Medical Library.

[117] The Annual Report on Mental Hospitals in the United Provinces for the Year 1939, NAI.

[118] Niall McCrae, '"A Violent Thunderstorm": Cardiazol Treatment in British Mental Hospitals', *History of Psychiatry*, vol. 17, no. 1 (2006): 68.

them in India.[119] Dhunjibhoy though made an extensive use of cardio-zol therapy for his patients.

Eric Cunningham Dax attempted to induce fits by using ammonium chloride in 1940 at the Netherne Mental Hospital, England. Niall McCrae has remarked that 'Dax (1940) tried ammonium chloride at Netherne, but although well tolerated the fits were weak'.[120] However, ammonium chloride became a good and cheap substitute for other drugs during World War II. As the Report for the Mental Hospitals of the United Provinces for the Year 1940 noted, 'At the Mental Hospital, Agra, Intravenous injections of Ammonium Chloride solutions have given excellent result[s] in the treatment of Schizophrenia. It provided a cheap substitute for Cardiazol which cannot be now obtained due to War.'[121] The Punjab Mental Hospital Report for the Year 1941 stated, 'The chief treatment for mental disorders done in the hospital is with Cardiazol, Ammonium Chloride, and Sulphosin. These treatments were carried out with encouraging results.'[122] These techniques continued to be used along with ECT in independent India. Electricity was used for the first time by the Italian neuro-psychiatrist Ugo Cerletti to induce fits in 1937. It soon became a viable and effective method for calming patients suffering from mental illness.

According to Ernst, Dhunjibhoy had ordered an ECT machine as early as 1939.[123] The ECT machine was subsequently introduced in the Agra Mental Hospital in 1945.[124] Ernst argues,

> Psychiatrists in British India during the 1920s, 1930s and 1940s—while working within the wider framework (and the constraints) of colonial politics and racial discrimination—used at the same time as their refer-ence points for clinical excellence the professional developments on the

[119] Ernst, 'Practising "Colonial" or "Modern" Psychiatry', 94.

[120] McCrae, 'Cardiazol Treatment in British Mental Hospitals', 80.

[121] The Annual Report of the Mental Hospital of the Punjab for the Year 1940, National Medical Library.

[122] The Annual Report of the Mental Hospital of the Punjab for the Year 1941, National Medical Library.

[123] Ernst, 'Practising "Colonial" or "Modern" Psychiatry', 99.

[124] The Annual Report on the Mental Hospitals in the United Provinces for the Year 1945, NAI.

international scene. Paying attention to doctors's international links and networks, and their knowledge and application of theories and treatments promulgated in the wider world, points us beyond the narrow confines of the 'colonial'.[125]

Ernst's analysis is based on her study of the Ranchi Indian Mental Hospital. Her conclusions cannot be generalized as regional specificities have to be recognized and contextualized. The asylums in the Punjab and Uttar Pradesh did not undergo advancement and cannot be regarded as 'modern', especially when compared to the Ranchi Mental Hospital. They at best were providers of shelter, food, and some therapeutics and at worst were overcrowded institutions lacking proper facilities for care and treatment of the insane.

***

Lunatic asylums were hierarchical organizations that contained different strata and groups having varied aspirations and separate identities. The 'thick narrative' has helped in corroborating ideas and experiences, research and practice, self and society, and displacement and identity. The dynamics of colonialism, institutionalisation, and human agency to some extent have been explored. The staff sometimes worked in harmony with each other but at other times clashed. The logistics of colonial asylum architecture were aligned to the key ideas of segregation, sanctification, and control. It has been contended that institutional structures were based upon mundane experiences. The bureaucracy that governed them was not a monolithic entity. A close reading of the archival material offers insights into official attitudes and should be considered significant for writing social histories of the people who lived and worked (staff and inmates) in these institutions. These structures evolved and devolved over the century. The taxonomies of madness reflect racial attitudes of the officials. Nonetheless, by the twentieth century and with more advances being made into the understanding of the human mind, categories and views informing psychiatric diseases became more 'medicalized'. Intellectual networks, international links,

---

[125] Ernst, 'Practising "Colonial" or "Modern" Psychiatry', 82.

and exchange of knowledge changed the ways in which madness was being understood in India and abroad. The flow of knowledge, infra-structure, and also technology often took more time to reach colonies such as India. Delay also depended on the regional variations, individual interests of the Superintendents, and infrastructural goals of the colonial state. It may be concluded that while the architecture and infrastructure (in some ways) of most asylums necessarily remained 'archaic' because of the financial exigencies of colonialism, there was a definite but slow change in terms of 'therapeutics of madness'.

3 Everyday Histories

Life inside the Asylum Walls

The first step towards recovery is taken when they can be induced to occupy themselves in some way, and the benefit both to themselves and coincidently to the institution is incalculable.[1]

T
he routinized lives of the inmates revolved around 'employment and amusement', 'diet and space', 'reform and reward', and 'resistance and adjustment'. The trope of the mundane provides a microscopic lens to delve deeper into the banal social lives of inmates behind the asylum walls. Work was emphasized for its therapeutic value but profits were central in order to make asylums self-sufficient. Work, in fact, became the yardstick by which a patient's recovery was measured,

[1] The Annual Report of the Lunatic Asylum of the Punjab for the Year 1902, National Medical Library.

and insanity was conceptualized as curable or incurable. An investigation into diet and recreation patterns helps construct the social history of psychiatry in colonial India. The complex temporal and spatial materialities of everyday lives inside the asylum are studied here in order to comprehend the role played by various actors and discern how authority was constantly reordered and redefined. It would also provide evidence of the connections between the effort to enforce discipline on the life of inmates and the problems related to the working of the colonial asylums. This would help to unravel the official world view and its zeal for reform that shaped the asylum's inner life.

Routine, Work, and Discipline

Moral management was pioneered by Philippe Pinel, a French physician whose acts of freeing the insane at the Saltpetriere and Bicetre have been regarded as a key moment in the history of madness. It was propounded that madness had to be disciplined by exercising moral control over the insane. Their willpower and self-discipline had to displace restraints of all sorts. Pinel's notions about moral management were employed in England by Samuel Tuke at the Retreat at York, which was an asylum for the insane that gained repute for the humane treatment of the mad. However, it was Robert Gardener Hill who introduced total non-restraint for the first time at the Lincoln County Asylum.

John Conolly popularized the principles of moral management and the non-restraint movement. He was the Superintendent of the Hanwell asylum, the largest public asylum in England. Conolly paid attention to minute details of asylum life. Andrew Scull has pointed out that 'Conolly was among the first to insist that, for the alienist, everything that occurred within an institution was relevant to cure, and in consequence nothing could be safely delegated into lay hands'.[2] In his work *The Construction and Government of Lunatic Asylums and Hospitals for*

---

[2] Andrew Scull, 'A Victorian Alienist: John Conolly, FRCP, DCL (1794–1866)', in *The Anatomy of Madness: Essays in the History of Psychiatry, People and Ideas*, vol. 1, edited by W. F. Bynum, Roy Porter, and Michael Shephard (London: Tavistock Publications, 1985), 134.

the Insane, Conolly provided elaborate details regarding the functioning and construction of asylums. Time was an important factor in determining asylum regimen and for handling insanity. Conolly stated that 'great regularity of hours tends much to break the monotony of private as well as public asylum, and should be strictly attended to. Everything should be performed or appointed or ready at the appointed hours and the tediousness of waiting entirely unknown, as it always leads to complains and irregularities.'[3] He believed regularity would break the monotony of the lives of patients and exert firmness. Control was exerted or restored through the regulation of rhythms of everyday life. The practitioners of moral management gave due importance to time and regarded the time management system to be therapeutic.

Contemporary accounts of Indian asylums are replete with examples of the strict regimentation of everyday routine. The Civil Surgeon of the Delhi asylum, Dr Taylor pointed out:

> The whole of the inmates are awoke at about sunrise and are taken out. They go to the latrine and have a smoke if they like, and they go to their work. They have their breakfast at 10 am and rest till about 3; after 3 they go out to work again till 5; then they are bathed and washed, and then have their dinner; after dinner they are talking and smoking till sunset or dark, when they go to bed. They are treated with greatest kindness.[4]

Routine, on the one hand, allowed entrenchment of authority and, on the other hand, it instilled a sense of discipline in the everyday lives of the inmates and the staff. The notions of routine were integrated with the idea of labour. Waltraud Ernst has remarked,

> These accounts describe the daily routines of the institutions in almost idyllic terms—the narrative resembling descriptions of prestigious places in England well known for their decidedly humane approach. Although their veracity may be doubted, they can be interpreted as representing

---

[3] John Conolly, *The Construction and Government of Lunatic Asylums and Hospitals for the Insane* (London: John Churchill, 1846), 77.

[4] The Annual Report of the Lunatic Asylums of the Punjab for the Year 1873, NAI.

part of the rhetoric in which the medical professionals themselves pre-
ferred to represent or legitimise their work to the outside world.[5]

Historically, in the West it was with the emergence of Protestantism
that the ethic of work became crucial. Sloth became a sin par excellence.
Foucault has argued that in order to chastise and discipline deviants,
the notion of 'labour' became imperative. In this sense, houses of correction were economic institutions—a solution for economic problems.
Private entrepreneurs used the labour of inmates of asylums for their
own profit.[6] Foucault asserts, 'In Paris several attempts were made to
transform the buildings of Hopital General into factories.'[7] James H.
Mills has looked at the issue of labour in the context of the Indian lunatic asylum. He observes, 'Work was central to the asylum regime and
the inmates were put to a range of tasks in the asylums of India, from
attending to the farms established within the asylum walls to perform-
ing maintenance around the asylum and even to participating in cottage
industry processes such as spinning and weaving.'[8]

The discourse on 'lazy natives' reinforced the notion that 'natives' have
to be 'civilized' through labour. The emphasis on work (and thrift) should
be seen against the backdrop of a longer process that was triggered by
industrialization and the changing conception of time. E. P. Thompson
in his well-known article 'Time, Work-Discipline and Industrial
Capitalism' charts out the development of time, work, and discipline.[9]
He postulates that from 'the spread of clocks in the fourteenth century to

[5]   Waltraud Ernst, 'The Establishment of "Native Lunatic Asylums" in Early
Nineteenth Century British India,' in *Studies in Indian Medical History*, edited
by G. Jan Meulenbeld and Dominik Wujastyk (Delhi: Motilal Banarsidass,
2001), 16.

[6]   Foucault, *Madness and Civilization*, 49.

[7]   Foucault, *Madness and* Civilization, 49.

[8]   James H. Mills, '"More Important to Civilize Than Subdue"? Lunatic
Asylums, Psychiatric Practice and Fantasies of "the Civilizing Mission" in British
India, 1858–1900', in *Colonialism as a Civilizing Mission: Cultural Ideology
in British India*, edited by Harald Fischer-Tine and Michael Mann (London:
Anthem South Asian Studies, 2004), 186–7.

[9]   E. P. Thomson, 'Time, Work-Discipline and Industrial Capitalism', *Past
and Present*, vol. 38, no.1 (1967): 56–97.

the Elizabethan age, the notions of time had not only emerged but also led to an advancement of morality related to work ethic.[10] By the beginning of the nineteenth century, the ideas about time, work, and discipline had become rigid. Thompson states that 'in all these ways—by the division of labour; the supervision of labour; fines; bells and clocks; money incentives; preachings and schoolings; the suppression of fairs and sports—new labour habits were formed, and a new time-discipline was imposed.'[11] He states that ideas of time and discipline were internalized by labourers and at times the process took several generations.[12] Thus, the poor were induced to work hard and develop industrious habits by the moralists and the Methodists. In India the responsibility of inculcating the 'work ethic' lay on the shoulders of the colonial state. Thompson asserts that the colonized were regarded as 'indolent and childlike'. He points out, for instance, that in the early years of the growth of Bombay cotton mills serious attempts were made to make labourers conscious about time and regularity.[13]

The 'dangerous' and the 'curable' were considered somewhat fitter to perform labour in the asylums than the 'incurables'. From early on there was a clear emphasis on the employment of patients. The Annual Return of the Insane Hospitals at Delhi, Bareilly, and Baneres for the Year 1853 emphasized the need for space for 'outdoor employment and amusement of the patients'.[14] By the late nineteenth century, the turnover of annual profits had become a special feature of the annual reports of the Indian lunatic asylums. A regimented routine was crucial in order to enforce the productivity of these so-called philanthropic institutions. In the context of the Bombay asylums, Sarah Ann Pinto argues that 'the colonial government in asylum treatment practices reinforced capitalist principles'.[15] In other words, the asylum acted like a small-scale cottage

[10] Thomson, 'Time, Work-Discipline and Industrial Capitalism': 56–7.

[11] Thomson, 'Time, Work-Discipline and Industrial Capitalism': 90–1.

[12] Thomson, 'Time, Work-Discipline and Industrial Capitalism': 90.

[13] Thomson, 'Time, Work-Discipline and Industrial Capitalism': 91–3.

[14] The Annual Return of the Insane Hospitals at Delhi, Bareilly and Benares for the Year 1853, E/4/ 833, British Library.

[15] Sarah Ann Pinto, 'Shackled Bodies, Unchained Minds: Lunatic Asylums in Bombay Presidency, 1793–1921', unpublished doctoral thesis (Wellington: Victoria University of Wellington, 2017), 104.

industry that aimed at self-sufficiency but attempts were also made to market the products made within the asylum walls. The Government of the North-Western Provinces and Oudh informed the Surgeon General of the province that 'all the asylums now manufacture a large share of their own clothing and bedding. This industry is somewhat new one in the North Western Provinces, so that one may hope that before long they will be able to supply the whole of their requirements of this kind'.[16]

G. F. W. Ewens, the Superintendent in Charge of the Punjab asylum wrote in the Triennial Report for the Years 1906–8:

> Though the manufactures carried on in the male asylum are primarily for its actual maintenance requirements, a small gang of men in excess of those so required, is employed on making munj matting for which there is great demand, far in excess indeed of what can be turned out were more men available, while others cut the grass growing on the asylum land in the summer which sells readily, and a profit of some Rs. 2,831, Rs. 2,908, Rs. 1,041 in the three years, respectively, was made in this way.[17]

The inmates performed a variety of tasks. They worked in the garden, cooked food, weaved blankets, and even cultivated land. Gender-based division of labour was prevalent. Women were occupied in spinning, weaving, cleaning, and cooking. Men were employed in manufacturing, cleaning, cultivating land, and work related to dairy farming. A look at the asylum statistics of employment and profit would allow us to further understand the way in which the system worked. The Report on the Lunatic Asylums in the North-Western Provinces and Oudh for the Year 1893 provides us with a following information:

Table 3.1 reflects attempts made by the authorities not only to show the rates of employment but also to record the efforts put in to engage the lunatics in useful work. This was necessary to justify the existence of these institutions.

---

[16] From the Government of the North Western Provinces and Oudh to the Surgeon General, Home Dept./Medical Branch, File No. 7–10, September 1894, NAI.

[17] The Triennial Report on the Lunatic Asylum in the Punjab for the Years 1906, 1907, and 1908, National Medical Library.

Table 3.1   The Rate of Employment of the Inmates

	Mean Population			Average Employed		
	1891	1892	1893	1891	1892	1893
Bareilly	318	325	300	132	136	87
Benares	293	281	267	111	90	86
Agra	211	214	218	49	49	110
Lucknow	184	201	207	95	102	118
Total	1,006	1,023	1,013	389	379	401

Note: The discrepancy in the calculation of total numbers existed in the asylum records.
Source: Annual Report of the Lunatic Asylums of the North-Western Provinces and Oudh for the Year 1893.

By the beginning of the twentieth century, a system of rewards was formalized. Inmates were not only given incentives in the form of additional allowance of food but monetary rewards were also offered to maintain the stability of the labour force. The Inspector General of Civil Hospitals, Bengal, wrote to the Secretary of the Government of Bengal,

> [This] system is in the force in the Dullanda and Patna Asylums. At the former a sum of Rs. 2 is distributed every month to two such lunatics one of whom is a good weaver and the other a good worker in the store godowns. The superintendents say that the system has been successful in encouraging lunatics to work. At Patna one rupee is at present drawn from the treasury and distributed among the hardworking and well-behaved lunatics, who spend the amount in buying sweets, fruits,etc., for themselves.[18]

Experiments with new forms of crops and products for marketing were also not uncommon. Dr Scriven, Superintendent of the Lahore asylum, noted in the Annual Report for the asylum:

> A small number are employed in manufactures which have never been very profitable in this asylum ... the following articles have been

[18] System of Rewarding Hard-Working and Well-Behaved Lunatics in Lunatic Asylum, Home Dept./Medical Branch, File No. 52–63, September 1901, NAI.

made:—188 blankets, 276¼ yards garrah cloth, 16 darrees, 7 seers 1 chattak newar, 54 reed chicks, 113 kilchee as kets, a maund 7 seers cotton thread, 17 yards doossuttee cloth, 8 moonj pardahs and 38 seers 3 chattaks munj ropes and twine.[19]

In Delhi the land near the lunatic asylum was reclaimed and crops were grown through the efforts of the inmates. Dr Fairweather wrote in 1879:

> The lunatics have been employed in the same way as last year. Their heaviest piece of work has been reclaiming the waste land belonging to the asylum. This was begun about two years ago, and two third of the field have now been trenched to a depth of 3 feet: and 2,360 cubic feet of large stone have been taken out of it during the year. The crop off this ground fetched Rs 44 during the hot weather and it is now being planted with tobacco, which it is hoped will bring a considerable sum.[20]

From this period onwards manufacture and hard labour became an integral part of life of the Delhi Lunatic Asylum.

A huge dairy farm was maintained at the Bareilly asylum. As the Annual Report of the North-Western Provinces for the Year 1891 noted:

> This important farm, which was started at the close of 1890, and is separately reported on, has, under the able management of Dr. Anderson, proved an unqualified success. On 31st December 1890 the stock, excluding calves, consisted of 69 cows and 4 buffaloes, which supplied the whole of the milk necessary for the Station Hospital and for Officers' Mess, 1st Hants Regiment. The surplus milk and butter were sold to individual purchasers, the balance sheet showing a net profit at the close of the year of Rs. 4008. It is probable that during 1892 the debt of the Military Department will be paid off, when the net receipts will form part of Provincial revenues.[21]

---

[19] The Annual Report of the Lunatic Asylums of the Punjab for the Year 1877, NAI.

[20] The Annual Report of the Lunatic Asylums of the Punjab for the Year 1879, NAI.

[21] The Annual Report of the Lunatic Asylums of the of the North Western Provinces and Oudh for the Year 1891, NAI.

These experiments at times met with success but occasionally failed. The dairy farm was closed down in 1908 due to high mortality rates among the cattle.[22] However, what remained consistent was the effort to make these institutions as profitable as possible.

Jennifer Laws has analysed Western notions about madness and the therapeutics of work. Her research spans the period from the nineteenth century to the twenty-first century. Laws points out that it was the moral management system that emphasized the significance of work and its related efficaciousness for curing insanity. Samuel Tuke in the York Retreat promoted employment of the insane for inducing recovery. Laws rightly remarks that 'moral therapy rested on a mixed philosophical heritage of Enlightenment faith in reason, burgeoning capitalist rational self-interest and (at the York Retreat) the Quaker ethics of prudence and self-control'.[23] Laws states that work, however, was not the sole basis of cure at the York Retreat. Rather, holistic organization of time based on the principles of 'work, rest and worship' was the cornerstone on which notions about cure rested.[24] She further notes,

> Professional organization of 'occupational therapy' did not begin until the mass return of shell-shocked soldiers at the end of the First World War, and the term 'occupational therapy' was not coined until 1914 at a professional meeting in New York. The movement arrived in Britain a decade later, when Scottish-born Margaret Fulton became Britain's first qualified occupational therapist at the Aberdeen Royal Asylum.[25]

The moral management system regarded work as being essential for restoring sanity. Occupational therapy, which relied heavily on the work ethic, was also an answer to the war economy.

In the Indian context, asylums came to be visualized as institutions for profit earning and experimentation. In the absence of poor laws,

---

[22] The Annual Report of the Lunatic Asylum of the N. W. P. and Oudh for the Year 1900, and the Triennial Report on the Lunatic Asylum in the United Provinces for the Years 1906, 1907, and 1908, NAI.

[23] Jennifer Laws, 'Crackpots and Basket-Cases: A History of Therapeutic Work and Occupation', *History of the Human Sciences*, vol. 24, no. 2 (2011): 67.

[24] Laws, 'Crackpots and Basket-Cases': 68.

[25] Laws, 'Crackpots and Basket-Cases': 69.

asylums in India became substitutes for institutions for poor relief as throughout the nineteenth century asylums were peopled by the poor. According to Ewens:

> In some of the cases their insanity has for one of its symptoms the utter refusal to do anything whatsoever, but in all the first step towards recovery is taken when they can be induced to occupy themselves in some way, and the benefit both to themselves and coincidently to the institution is incalculable. It would, of course, be impossible to work the asylum with its present staff and at its present cost without a large number of its inmates being employed in its actual maintenance, and thus the cooking, cleaning, sweeping, washing, &c., employs a good number. The large garden also provides an excellent and healthy form of labour for many. ... Nothing is more striking than to note the gradual improvement in a man once induced to labour, or to see an acute maniac raving, shouting, gesticulating, tearing everything within his reach, soften down, after a few days' violent exercise at mulling blankets, into a quiet and reasonable patient.[26]

Work became a key principle for the treatment of the insane. Work was the index by which a patient's recovery was measured. Patients who had the ability to work were declared 'improved' or 'cured'. Much before the birth of occupational therapy, professionalization of 'insane' labour occurred in the Indian asylums. This vocational economy of asylums sustained the asylum's system throughout the colonial period. Ernst, more recently, assesses labour in the Indian asylums and she argues that 'institutions clearly profited from the products of patient work, in particular domestic chores that did not find monetary expression in accounts. However, mental hospitals did not produce big enough monetary gains to induce the colonial administration to maintain these institutions on profit grounds alone.'[27] There is no doubt that the colonial administration did not earn enough to maintain the institutions on profits alone. But there was a workhouse-ish fervour to push more and more patients to engage

---

[26] The Annual Report of the Lunatic Asylum of the Punjab for the Year 1902, National Medical Library.

[27] Waltraud Ernst, 'Useful Both for the Patients as well as to the State: Patient Work in the Colonial Mental Hospitals in South Asia, c. 1818–1948', in Work, Psychiatry and Society, c.1750–2015, edited by Waltraud Ernst (Manchester: Manchester University Press, 2016), 121.

in labour. It rose from the exegencies of colonial financial management that called for self-sufficiency of such institutions as they were regarded as burdensome. The government left only a handful of incurables and senseless patients alone. Therefore, it can be argued that 'from clothing to bedding and from diet to treatment nothing was "free of charge"; since the inmates had to actively work to run these institutions.'[28]

Daily Diet

Proper sleep, healthy labour, and nutritious diet were considered to be the main principles of moral treatment. Samuel Tuke in his book *Description of the Retreat* underlined the fact that in the York Retreat food was given three times a day. It included milk, bread, porridge, animal food, bread, and beer. Tuke believed that diet was an imperative part of treatment and he asserted that diet in the Retreat was 'more liberal than judicious.'[29] Robert Gardnier Hill, the Superintendent of the Lincoln Lunatic Asylum was a great proponent of the non-restraint movement. He, like other advocates, averred that 'generous diet implies a daily supply of animal food with different vegetables, varied as much as possible, and supplemented from time to time with fish, fruit, and farinaceous compounds—well cooked and well served adequate proportions, so that no one at the conclusion of the repast shall be able to say that he has not had enough.'[30] Leonard D. Smith has researched on early nineteenth-century asylums in England and states that 'asylum food exemplified the interface between principles of economic management and those of curative treatment. With the improvement of physical health deemed an essential element in the restoration of mental health, patients' diet was a central part of the treatment armoury.'[31]

[28] For details, see Shilpi Rajpal, 'Colonial Psychiatry in Mid-Nineteenth Century: The James Clark Enquiry', *South Asia Research*, vol. 35. no. 1, (2015): 77.

[29] Samuel Tuke, *Description of the Retreat: An Institution Near York for Insane Persons of the Society of Friends* (York, England: W. Alexander, 1813), 129.

[30] Robert Gardiner Hill, *Lunacy: Its Past and Its Present* (London: Longman, Green, 1870), 69.

[31] Leonard D. Smith, *'Cure, Comfort and Safe Custody': Public Lunatic Asylums in Early Nineteenth-Century England* (London: Leicester University Press, 1999), 164–5.

The moral management system had only a few tools that included control of the environment surrounding the lunatics and the use of therapeutics. The patient, therefore, had to be disciplined through a few available viable means. Diet remained at the heart of the system. Food helped in controlling the behaviour of the inmates and it also became a significant way of expressing care and kindness. A regulated diet formed an essential part of asyum life. The Code of Regulations stated in 1833 that 'the diet for patients under the medical treatment will, of course, be varied according to the circumstances of their several cases; and, in particular instances, such extra articles, as much to be considered proper, will be allowed, under the sanction of superintending surgeon'.[32] This power of a Superintendent to provide extra food to patients was not clearly charted. Food, therefore, became a tool to punish or reward patients in the asylum.

The asylum reports are sagas of generosity shown by the colonial state. C. M. Smith, the Superintendent of the Lahore asylum, pointed out in the Annual Report for the Year 1868 that 'every attention has been paid to the diet; the rations are inspected and passed by the deputy superintendent, both in their raw and cooked state. The meals have been issued at regular hours twice a day, and the same order and decency of conduct during meals has been enforced'.[33] Andrew Scull points out that somatic treatments played a crucial role in the history of psychiatry. He remarks that 'therapeutics, the translation of abstract knowledge into socially acceptable recipes for intervention and practical action, necessarily remains close to the heart of the medical enterprise'.[34]

Food was given twice a day. Breakfast was served at 9 a.m. and supper at 5 p.m. Contrary to the suggestions of pioneers of giving three meals, only two meals were offered at strictly regulated timings in the Indian asylums during the nineteenth century. These meals consisted of vegetables, rice, wheat, milk, and ghee (clarified butter). Mutton

[32] *Code of Regulations for the Medical Department of the Presidency of Fort St. George* (Madras: Printed at the Asylum Press, 1833), 169.

[33] The Annual Report of the Lunatic Asylums of the Punjab for the Year 1868, NAI.

[34] Andrew Scull, 'Somatic Treatments and the Historiography of Psychiatry', *History of Psychiatry*, vol. 5, no. 1 (1994): 2.

was issued twice a week in summer, and in winter three or four times a week.[35] Milk, ghee, and rum were usually given to convalescents. Fruits and sweetmeats were given on festive occasions.[36] The diet was given in limited quantities. Men were given 10 chittacks[37] while women were given 8 chittacks. Throughout the nineteenth century, the quantity and the quality of diet were not standardized. It depended on the Superintendents' and the local government officials' understanding of how to qualify and quantify the diet of the asylum's inmates. Therefore, the expenses related to diet differed from one asylum to the other.

The diet regimen came under scrutiny only if the mortality rates were high or the cost of food was exorbitant. Also, ex-officio visitors sometimes made criticisms and highlighted the problems. The Annual Returns of the asylums in Delhi, Benares, and Bareilly for 1849 stated that 'the great mortality at Benares was in a great degree owning to insufficient dietary [sic]'.[38] The conditions in the Delhi asylum were not rectified completely and the asylum came under governmental scrutiny again in the year 1871. The visitors who were the Inspector General of Hospitals and the Inspector General of Jails highlighted the inadequacies and, among other complaints, an objection was made to the diet scale. They noted that the food given to inmates was inadequate. Dr Taylor, the Superintendent in Charge of the Delhi asylum stated in the Annual Report for the Year 1872:

> Both Dr. Tresidder and Dr. Dallas [visitors] have recommended an increase in the quantity of ghee and salt, and that the rice and dall comprising Friday's diet from eight to ten chittack. In this I quite agree, and I have given the order for increase in anticipation of its sanction. I am of the opinion, after having most carefully watched the cases for last eight

[35] The Annual Report of the Lunatic Asylums of the Punjab for the Year 1870, NAI.

[36] The Annual Report of the Lunatic Asylums of the Punjab for the Year 1870, NAI.

[37] In Bengal, 1 chittack was a unit of mass which was equivalent to 5 tolas (1 tola is 11.66 grams) or 1/16th seer (1 seer is approximately 0. 93310 kilogramme).

[38] The Annual Returns of the Asylums in Delhi, Benares and Bareilly for the Year 1849, E/4/818, British Library.

months, and the death rate would be reduced by a more liberal dietary, I think the female ones should have as much as the males.[39]

Statistics showed that the next year the mortality rate had dropped by a considerable degree. Nevertheless, the diet was barely sufficient as even after this limited increase, Dr Taylor remarked that he was 'anxious to be allowed to increase the diet of the lunatics.'[40] He also pointed out that women were given less food in comparison to men. For the next two years, Dr Taylor reiterated the urgent need to increase the diet scale of the female inmates. In the Annual Report for the Year 1874, Taylor had the following to say:

> The diet scale is the same as it was last year. I think that the women should have more food. I recommended last year that they should have the same quantity as the male. I understand that in the North-West Provinces the allowance of flour is 12 chittacks per diem for both male and female; here it is 10 chittack for the former and 8 for latter. This is not enough I fear, and the high death rate of the females, contrasted with the very small mortality among the males, renders me very anxious to be allowed to increase the amount of the former food. The women and men both complain of not having enough food, but I think, though the men both could and would eat more if they could get it, the women are only in absolute want of an increase.[41]

It was only after Dr Taylor's incumbency that the diet scale of females was increased from 8 to 10 chittacks.[42] Taylor disregarded men's complaints of 'not having enough food' and their diet remained unaltered.

Numerous attempts were made to economize expenditure in the lunatic asylums. The ramifications of this economizing drive had a serious effect on asylum food. The expenditure on food in asylums was

[39] The Annual Report of the Lunatic Asylums of the Punjab for the Year 1872, NAI.

[40] The Annual Report of the Lunatic Asylums of the Punjab for the Year 1873, NAI.

[41] The Annual Report of the Lunatic Asylums of the Punjab for the Year 1874, NAI.

[42] The Annual Report of the Lunatic Asylums of the Punjab for the Year 1875, NAI.

considered to be excessively high, especially when compared to that on food in the jails. J. C. Scriven, the Superintendent of the Lahore Lunatic Asylum was of the opinion that 'the food has been much more expensive than the jail food, as meat is supplied in small quantity every working day. We calculated some months ago that if the meat were cut out the food would cost nearly the same as the jail food.'[43] Such comparisons show how jails and asylums were invariably linked in the official discourse. This would have had an effect on determining the dietary scale of the asylums. The Superintendent in Charge of the Lahore asylum pointed out,

> On comparing the dietary of this Asylum with that of other establishments of the same kind in other parts of the country as well as with the dietary of Punjab jails, I discovered that the allowance of ghi and fatty matter was much smaller than in these. On representing this through the surgeon-general, Punjab, the allowance of ghi was raised from 1/5 chittak to 1/2 chittak per head during the colder months of November, December, January and February.[44]

The moral management movement preached kindness and humanity. An important principle of the system was that lunatics should be treated as patients and not as criminals. The practice of sending lunatics to jail was largely discarded in England. However, the ideals of the non-restraint movement were never practised in their totality in India. Lunatics were generally treated as ordinary criminals and insanity was virtually a criminal offence in colonial India. As W. Walker, the Officiating Surgeon, the Government of India, put it:

> It hardly needs to be pointed out that the vast majority of the lunatic confined in the asylums are paupers and criminal lunatics; and the first principle to lay down is that in all cases in which the pauper or criminal lunatic is in sound physical health, there is no need to treat him to any large extent differently in matters of diet, clothing & c. from one of the free population, or from prisoner in the same class of life in our jails.

[43] The Annual Report of the Lunatic Asylums of the Punjab for the Year 1878, NAI.

[44] The Annual Report of the Lunatic Asylums of the Punjab for the Year 1881, NAI.

It is no doubt difficult to draw the line in case of mental disease between a condition of sound and unsound physical health; but this is not so difficult as to necessitate that every pauper insane and every criminal lunatic in an asylum should be treated as a patient in hospital. If the lunatic or his friend can pay for his support, the case is different; but as long as he is a pauper in sound physical health there is no reason why he should live more luxuriously in a lunatic asylum than he would in his own house. This principle is acted upon in all European asylums for the insane.[45]

The monotony of the institution gave to food a special place in the lives of inmates. The officials were well aware of this fact and, therefore, used food to control the behaviour of inmates. Food items such as fruits and sweets and even stimulants such as tobacco and cigarettes were used to induce the lunatics to perform hard labour.[46] This approach of 'reward and punishment' was integral to the moral management system. Smith points out that in the English asylums 'patients "actively employed" in the asylum or its grounds received extra diet.'[47] The Superintendent in Charge of the Delhi asylum remarked in the context that 'on Sunday all are treated to either sweetmeats, or fruits in their season. This treat is looked forward by them, and in the cases of misbehavior it is withheld as a means of punishment.'[48] The Superintendent was setting an example by withdrawing food as a form of punishment. This policy of reward and punishment was monetzed by the beginning of the twentieth century when food items were replaced by monetary stipends.

Recreation

Recreation was considered to be therapeutic as various forms of entertainment broke the monotony of the patients and enabled inmates to

[45] Note by the Officiating Surgeon General with the Government of India, 24 August 1888. Expenditure in Lunatic Asylums in India, Home Dept./Medical, File No. 68–70, September 1888, NAI.

[46] The Triennial Report on the Lunatic Asylum in the Punjab for the Years 1912, 1913, and 1914, National Medical Library.

[47] Smith, 'Cure, Comfort and Safe Custody', 165.

[48] The Annual Report of the Lunatic Asylums of the Punjab for the Year 1875, NAI.

relax. Dolly MacKinnon argues that 'providing entertainment combated the effects of institutionalisation. Entertainment and recreation gave selected inmates normal experiences of the outside world "inside" the asylum walls'.[49] This section looks at the forms of recreation made available to inmates in north Indian asylums. Amusement was an essential part of the moral management system and, therefore, it was considered to be a part of the treatment regimen. Entertainment was provided to the inmates along the lines of 'race' and class. In the nineteenth century, European patients were provided with amenities of superior quality, whereas Indian patients were provided with inferior facilities. By the turn of the century, superior facilities were being provided to Indian inmates who could pay for them.

The James Clark Enquiry probing the conditions of the asylums was conducted, as we have noted, in 1868. Among the queries that it had was one pertaining to whether there was a dining room or recreational hall in the asylum. J. C Whishaw, the Civil Surgeon of the Cuttack asylum, responded with the answer: 'The patients dine—as almost all natives of Hindoostan dine—in the open air. When it rains they dine in a covered shed. There is no recreational hall'.[50] Many of the other Superintendents pointed out that they strategically used the work-shed as the dining floor. The question related to the recreational hall or space for recreation was raised again by Robert Harvey in 1899 and by Jameson in 1922.[51] Throughout the colonial period, recreational spaces were improvised by appropriating spaces intended for other purposes (work-shed, and such others), but rarely were built specifically for recreation.

[49] Dolly MacKinnon, '"Amusements Are Provided": Asylum Entertainment and Recreation in Australia and New Zealand c.1860–c.1945', in *Permeable Walls: Historical Perspectives on Hospital and Asylum Vistings*, edited by Graham Mooney and Jonathan Reinarz (New York: Rodopi, 2009), 268.

[50] Sir James Clark's Enquiry as to the Care and the Treatment of Lunatics, Home Dept./Public Branch, File No. 22–23, 19 December 1868, NAI.

[51] Sir James Clark's Enquiry; Plans for the New Central Asylum to Be Constructed at Lahore, Home Dept./Medical Branch, May 1899, Nos 66 to 85, NAI; Amendment of the Indian Lunacy Act (IV of 1912), So as to Provide the Change of Designation of Lunatic Asylums to Mental Hospitals, Home Dept./Jail Branch, 1922, File No. 88, NAI.

Entertainment was considered to be a significant part of the official regimen. Dr Fairweather, Superintendent in Charge of the Delhi asylum, noted, 'Every inducement is given to the lunatics to amuse themselves in any way they can, and for this purpose kites, toys, tom-toms, *sittars* are provided for those who care for them. The women have pet pigeons, rabbits and lambs; swings are erected for their amusement.'[52] A wide array of recreation was offered to the Indian and European patients. G. Hutheson, the Inspector General of Civil Hospitals of the North-Western Provinces and Oudh stated in the Annual Report of 1899:'Different sorts of games, musical instruments, etc., were provided for natives; and books, papers, etc., procured for the European lunatics. In Bareilly, one of the European female lunatics was allowed out of the asylum for exercise. On festivals sweetmeats, fruit and extra diet were issued. The general effect of such indulgences was beneficial.'[53] In this context, asylum records are also replete with derogatory and racial undertones. Charles Lodge Patch remarked, the 'medical superintendent before myself had endeavoured to interest their patients in games of various sorts but their efforts were frustrated by the naturally slothful temperament of their enegies.'[54] Inmates' inability to adjust themselves to the environment was regarded as slothful. The patient's recovery was, therefore, dependent on their ability to participate in the activities of the institution.

The insane were at times taken out for rides on special occasions. Dr Penny stated, 'I borrowed the Municipal carts and sent them in a general procession, all dressed in their best. They went to Ram lela and Dewallee in my presence, and it was delightful to see the sympathy they met with from the passer-by.'[55] Entertainers were hired to perform in the asylums. According to D. O'C. Raye, the Inspector General of Civil Hospitals, the Punjab asylum,

[52] The Annual Report of the Lunatic Asylums of the Punjab for the Year 1875, NAI.

[53] The Annual Report of the Lunatic Asylums of North Western Provinces and Oudh for the Year 1899, NAI.

[54] Charles J. Lodge Patch, 'Birth of a Hospital', unpublished, typescript account of the mental hospital in Lahore, Private Papers, Mss Eur F544, British Library, 267.

[55] The Annual Report of the Lunatic Asylums of the Punjab for the Year 1870, NAI.

The Superintendent of the Delhi Asylum mentions that, having had a small sum of money placed at his disposal by the Deputy Commissioner, and by some generous native gentlemen, he was able to give to such of the lunatics as were capable of enjoying it the amusement of a weekly nautch. He engaged a couple of bazár minstrels for this purpose. Dr. Dennys writes that he was much struck with the soothing influence which this native music seemed to have on some of the refractory and troublesome insanes; and he considers that the experiment was a success, not only by giving some enjoyment to a number of pitiable and unhappy lives, but also by having an actually beneficial effect on the mental state of some of the sufferers.[56]

Nautches (Indian dance and musical performances) were at times considered beneficial, but at other times were regarded as injurious to the mental health of the inmates. Ernst has pointed out that some officials considered these nautches as harmful.[57] The effects of nautches were debated but they were never banned at large. A report on the lunatic asylums of the United Provinces stated in the context that 'amusements of various sorts (performances by jugglers, acrobats, minstrels) and native entertainments were provided for the lunatics' on a regular basis.[58]

A number of physical activities such as various games and different forms of physical exercises including walks were also introduced. Exercise and other physical activities have been regarded as foundational for the treatment of insanity.[59] In the words of Ewens:

Some of the sane men have built themselves little praying platforms, and all are allowed to keep religious books; means for gymnastics are

[56] The Annual Report of the Lunatic Asylums of the Punjab for the Year 1897, National Medical Library.

[57] Waltraud Ernst, 'Institutions, People and Power: Lunatic Asylums in Bengal, c. 1800–1900', in *The Social History of Health and Medicine in Colonial India*, edited by Biswamoy Pati and Mark Harrison (London: Routledge, 2009), 144.

[58] The Triennial Report on the Lunatic Asylums of the United Provinces for the Years 1906, 1907, and 1908, NAI.

[59] Waltraud Ernst, 'Therapy and Empowerment, Coercion and Punishment, Historical and Contemporary Perspectiveson Work, Psychiatry and Society', in *Work, Psychiatry and Society, c.1750–2015*, edited by Waltraud Ernst (Manchester: Manchester University Press, 2016), 5.

provided though rarely used; a native paper is taken in, and in addition to various native games the asylum possesses a gramophone and magic lantern. Tobacco is amply provided, and at all the native festivals and at Christmas issues of 'sweet rice', fruit and sweetmeats are made, and native jugglers and rag-doll performers engaged. A sanctioned allowance of 10 rupees monthly is divided in rewards among the best workers and keenly appreciated, while there are facilities arranged with the contractor for spending this and any other private money their relatives may have provided them with. In short everything possible is done to make their existence as easy as possible and their surroundings pleasant, and it may reasonably be claimed that they are as comfortable as they can be made.[60]

Religious activities were encouraged and the inmates were allowed to practise the rituals of their respective religions. Further as discussed earlier, rewards were monetized by the beginning of the twentieth century. Opening of shops within the confines of asylum walls was a reflection of this increased amount of monetization. Such facilities allowed inmates to spend the money, but in order to buy items from the shop, they had to work hard or else they had to depend upon their relatives for monetary resources.

The forms of recreation underwent transformation between early and mid-twentieth century. G. Tate, the Inspector General of Civil Hospitals, noted in the Triennial Rreport of the United Provinces for the Years 1924–6:

> Recreation is also arranged for. Pachisi, satranj, cards, etc., are provided in every section. Sing songs with *dhols* and *manjiras* find great favour on Sundays while healthy and regular exercise is obtained by foot-ball, tennis and walking, etc. in the 'better class' section. The Fauji Akhbar, Vakil and Bharat-Mitra as well as books are purchased for the sections. Nautch-girls come round occasionally and visit all the sections singing and dancing in each.[61]

Since the 1930s the patients were taken out for motor rides. Charles Lodge Patch, the Superintendent of the Punjab hospital, was of the opinion

[60] The Triennial Report on the Lunatic Asylum of the Punjab for the Years 1906, 1907, and 1908, National Medical Library.

[61] The Triennial Report on the Mental Hospitals in the United Provinces for the Years 1924, 1925, and 1926, NAI.

that 'more than anything, the patients appreciate drives in the motor bus; but in spite of frequent renewals of spare parts, the bus is threatened with signs of a complete break-down, and the question of its renewal will have to be considered within the next year or two'.[62] Modernization occurred not only in forms of emulating new techniques of treatment and entertainment but also in adapting to 'class-based' arrangements. From the beginning of the twentieth century, the number of patients admitted in these asylums increased considerably. These patients belonged to the middle classes and a new set of arrangements was introduced to cater to their specific needs. Ernst observes that 'the British class system had its equivalent in the highly stratified Indian caste system, and in divisions made along lines of religious, cultural, regional and class affiliation'.[63]

The standards of the mental hospitals were improved by allowing a better arrangement for the class of paying patients. From the late 1920s onwards, electrification of the asylums had taken place. The Triennial Report for the Mental Hospitals in the United Provinces for 1936–8 lauded efforts for '[the] establishment of fiction library for patients ... [and the] provision of Radio sets'.[64] Most of the mental hospitals had a library. Charles Lodge Patch remaked that 'mental patients need lighter literature, so I bought several hundreds of volumes in English and in the vernacular'.[65] Moreover, 'at the Mental Hospital Agra the patients and the staff had formed teams in the year 1941 by the name of the Menthosp Club. These teams played several hockey and football matches with the local team'.[66] D. Clyde, the Inspector General of Civil Hospitals, Punjab, noted in the Annual Report for the Year 1945:

Certain games and articles for amusement are supplied to the patients. Patients are taken out [for] a walk daily in the morning and evening

[62] The Triennial Report on the Mental Hospitals in the United Provinces for the Years 1927, 1928, and 1929, NAI.

[63] Waltraud Ernst, 'Madness and Colonial Spaces British India, 1800–1947', in *Madness, Architecture and the Built Environment*, edited by Leslie Topp, James Moran, and Jonathan Andrews (London: Routledge, 2007), 220.

[64] The Triennial Report on the Mental Hospitals of the United Provinces for the Years 1936, 1937, and 1938, NAI.

[65] Patch, 'Birth of a Hospital', 268.

[66] The Annual Report on the Mental Hospitals of the Punjab for the Year 1945, NAI.

and are also taken to cinemas. Messrs. Mehra Brothers and Narain Dass of Lahore each continued to supply 7 gallons of petrol free of cost for the running of the bus of the hospital and the proprietors of the following cinemas showed their generosity by issuing free cinema passes to mental patients. 1. Nishat, 2. Palace, 3. Regent, 4. Prabhat, and 5. Ritz.[67]

The nature of amusement underwent change not just because of changes in technology but also due to the transformation that was occurring within and outside the walls of the asylum. Since the beginning of the twentieth century, numerous attempts were made to disseminate information about the asylums. The changing character of these mental hospitals attracted not only paying patients but also voluntary donations and help. According to C. C. Manifold, Inspector General of the Civil Hospitals of the United Province,

> [A] small concert is arranged fortnightly by the staff assisted by their friends which is much enjoyed by the inmates. A Christmas tree was provided and a special dinner and tea for the occasion. This year a donation of Rs. 40 was subscribed by members of the Telegraph department at Agra, and a tennis and badminton party with a string band helped considerably to make a bright and memorable occasion for the European inmates.[68]

In England, as well as in some other British settler colonies such as Australia, asylum balls were a common feature. Dolly MacKinnon suggests that 'entertainments forged important political and social links between the invited guests and the institution.'[69] In the Indian context, lavish balls were never part of the recreational plan but by the twentieth century the asylum walls became permeable as local communities, groups, and notable dignitaries of the city were expected to do voluntary work for these institutions. Recreation was a crucial part of everyday life

---

[67] The Annual Report of the Mental Hospital of the Punjab for the Year 1945, NAI.

[68] The Triennial Report on Lunatic Asylums of the United Provinces for the Years 1912, 1913, and 1914, NAI.

[69] MacKinnon, 'Asylum Entertainment and Recreation in Australia and New Zealand', 272.

in the asylums. It rejuvinated not only the inmates of the asylum but the staff as well.

Everyday Lives: Patients and Personnel

Erving Goffman in his work *Asylum* has pointed out that 'each grouping tends to conceive of the other in terms of narrow hostile stereotypes, staff often seeing inmates as bitter, secretive and untrustworthy, while inmates often see staff as condescending, highhanded and mean'.[70] He argues that people at the bottom of the hierarchy are usually more dissatisfied with their jobs and the ways of life than the high-handed officials who cherish their privileges and work. Thus, they would utilize their circumstances legitimately or illegitimately in order to meet their ends. Goffman calls these everyday adaptations involving 'unauthorized means' to meet 'unauthorized ends' *secondary adjustment*.[71] For Goffman, the *primary adjustment* is a process through which an individual transforms himself into a cooperator.[72] Goffman calls this the 'underlife' of the mental institution. This underlife could at times be marked by violence. In a volatile form, the inmates try to upset the structure whereas in a 'restrictive' form of life the inmates attempt to make small adjustments by subverting the regimes. It may be noted here that in the mental institutions, the subordinate staff and the patients were approximately at similar levels of hierarchy. They lived their underlives at individualistic as well as at the social levels. The staff could do this secondary adjustment secretively or with other selected members of the staff. They could also at times engage patients to meet their ends or the patients could assimilate with some members of the staff in order to fulfil their aims. These situations are much more feasible in the mental hospitals than in other institutions because of their isolated nature and drab way of life. This section tries to reconstruct the 'underlife' of the asylums in the colonial north Indian lunatic asylums. Goffman's hypothesis gives us an insight into the multiple layers of enmeshed lives of the patients and the staff.

---

[70] Erving Goffman, *Asylums: Essays on the Social Situation of Mental Patients and Other Inmates* (Chicago: Aldine, 1962), 7.

[71] Goffman, *Asylums*, 172.

[72] Goffman, *Asylums*, 172.

R. Charles Macwatt, the Inspector General of Civil Hospitals, Punjab, noted in the Annual Report for the Year 1918:

> There has been in 1917, one death from an overdose of opium in a criminal and there is strong reason to believe that the drug was self-administered owing to grief following the death of the man's wife. In this connection, it may be mentioned the great difficulty, nay, the impossibility of preventing the surreptitious entry of toxic drugs through the agency of the attendants and sweepers. Regular searches are conducted of all such leaving and entering the asylum, but it is obvious that small parcels such as these drugs readily escape detection.[73]

H. W. V. Cox, the Superintendent of the Punjab Lunatic Asylum, also had the same problem: 'In this connection it may be mentioned how futile our precautionary measures are for preventing the entry of toxic drugs through the agency of asylum servants, when it is pointed out how easy it is to introduce such drugs by simply throwing packets over the enclosure walls.'[74] These examples point towards a high level of complicity existing between the inmates and the attendants. Hemp and other narcotic substances were considered to be the major causes of insanity. Smuggling of these items was a combined attempt made by the subordinate groups to subvert the authorities and the discipline sought to be imposed in the asylums. These attempts formed part of the indirect confrontations that must have occurred at several levels. They largely went unnoticed as they were not considered worthy of mentioning in the annual reports or official memos.

There were other ways through which the patients and the staff subverted the everyday structures. Dr Fairweather of the Delhi asylum pointed out in the Annual Report for 1875, 'I regret I cannot report favourably about the subordinate establishment. The assistant matron, the cook and a keeper have been discharged for stealing the lunatics food, and several of burkanzadas [armed guards] and keepers have been fined or dismissed for carelessness and harsh treatment of the lunatics under

---

[73] The Annual Report of the Lunatic Asylum of the Punjab for the Year 1918, National Medical Library.

[74] The Annual Report on the Lunatic Asylum in the Punjab for the Year 1921, National Medical Library.

their charge.'[75] G. Ross, the Superintendent of the Delhi asylum, mentioned in the Annual Report for the Year 1880:

> A new and very respectable man has been appointed in place of Salik Ram whom I dismissed, as he was arrested by the police on a charge of appropriating a piece of timber, the property of Government. He was altogether an ill-conducted man, and the asylum is well rid of him. I was obliged to prosecute the malli for being found in the female quarters at night, and also to make some changes among the warders. The visitors met once a month to inspect the asylum and to consider releases and admissions.[76]

James C. Scott has pointed out that subordinate groups often use 'everyday forms of resistance'.[77] For him, when these groups cannot take political action they resort to everyday forms of resistance that include

> such acts as foot-dragging, dissimulations, false compliance, feigned igno-rance, desertion, pilfering, smuggling, poaching, arson, slander, sabotage, surreptitious assault and murder, anonymous threats, and so on. These techniques, for the most part quite prosaic, are the ordinary means of class struggle. They are the techniques of 'first resort' in those common historical circumstances in which open defiance is impossible or entails mortal danger.[78]

Stealing objects or having sexual relationships with inmates were inte-gral to the daily acts of defiance that were resorted to by the subordinate staff in the absence of direct action.

The patients resisted against attempts to force them to lead a dehumanized existence by refusing to eat food or wearing clothes.[79]

---

[75] The Annual Report of the Lunatic Asylums of the Punjab for the Year 1875, NAI.

[76] The Annual Report of the Lunatic Asylums of the Punjab for the Year 1880, NAI.

[77] James C. Scott, 'Everyday Forms of Resistance', *Copenhagen Journal of Asian Studies*, vol. 67, no. 4 (1989): 33.

[78] The Annual Report of the Lunatic Asylums of the Punjab for the Year 1887, NAI.

[79] Pinto regards clothing as a part of the treatment and as a form of estab-lishing authority over the inmates. For details, see Pinto, 'Shackled Bodies', 95–6.

The Superintendent in Charge of the Delhi asylum, T. E. L. Bate, remarked in the Annual Report for the Year 1887, 'Many of the lunatics throw off their clothing and bedding, and in this way expose themselves to chill which is of course calculated to produce disease. Again many are very capricious and refuse their food from time to time. In such cases, although artificial feeding is resorted to, their health suffers.'[80] Pinto points out that 'asylum staff commonly resorted to force-feeding patients and even employed patients in restraining other patients who refused food.'[81] She argues that refusal of food was regarded as a sign of their mental illness. Forced feeding was, therefore, regarded as a way of curing patients. C. Manifold, the Inspector General of the Civil Hospitals, wrote in the Triennial Report of the United Provinces for 1909–11: 'It was a case of acute mania, the patient being constantly excited. He was very destructive, tearing up and throwing out of his cell the whole of his clothing and bedding. He contracted pneumonia from exposure, and being in a very run-down condition soon succumbed to the disease.'[82] These forms of resistance should be regarded as a definite pattern of everyday survival. Adjustments were a two-way road, where sometimes the patients adjusted, at other times the authorties atoned.

Escape and suicide were other common ways of defiance. H. J. Maynard, the Junior Secretary to Government, Punjab, pointed out:

> It has been alleged that criminals purposely feign insanity in the hope of being committed to the Lahore Asylum, whence escapes are known to be facilitated by structural defects which make the buildings unsuitable for the confinement of even ordinary lunatics. Whether the statement that criminals feign lunacy for the purpose indicated be true or not it is a curious coincidence that quite recently the number of escapes from the Asylum have been unprecedented. It will be observed that there were no less than 10 escapes [in] 1897 and several have already occurred during the current year. The escape of criminal lunatics is serious, and in view of the fact that reports in respect to watch and ward were unsatisfactory.[83]

---

80 Scott, 'Everyday Forms of Resistance', 33.

81 Pinto, 'Shackled Bodies', 98.

82 The Triennial Report on the Lunatic Asylums in the United Provinces for the Years 1909, 1910, and 1911, NAI.

83 H. J. Maynard, the Junior Secretary to Government, Punjab Proceedings of the Hon'ble the Lieutenant Governor of the Punjab, in the Home (Medical

Mills points out that Indians often had hidden agendas and they made use of the asylum space according to their needs. Criminals used the asylum in order to escape harsh treatment and to subsequently run away from the asylums. The inmates, when they felt repressed, often resorted to suicide. The Superintendent of the Lahore asylum stated:

> Suicide was absolutely unknown from the opening of the asylum up to 1906, when a woman utterly without warning hanged herself by her clothing during the night and a man a few days later followed her example. Then in 1908 a man suddenly hanged himself with a strip of blanketing and two others followed suit at short intervals. It is difficult to see how such occurrences can be prevented especially in the winter; even with the most vigilant attendants and none of those here answer that description, every man cannot possibly be always under supervision and short of depriving them literally of all clothing they cannot fail to have facilities for effecting their purpose.[84]

Strict vigilance was not adequate to prevent suicides. Suicide was sometimes a result of melancholy but it was also frequently the 'last resort' against a degraded existence. Suicidal patients formed an important category among the incarcerated patients, but official reports only highlight cases of patients who had committed suicide, with there being few details of patients with suicidal tendencies.[85]

Illustrative cases of survival also come to the fore. According to Manifold: 'In 1911 one death was due to heart failure following on old age. The patient had been 37 years in confinement and was 60 years old when he died.'[86] These survivors had not only made these alien places

---

and Sanitary), The Annual Report of the Lunatic Asylum of the Punjab for the Year 1898, National Medical Library.

[84] The Triennial Report on the Lunatic Asylum in the Punjab for the Years 1906, 1907, and 1908, National Medical Library.

[85] There are some interesting works on suicide and suicidal patients in England. For details, see A. Shepherd and D. Wright, 'Madness, Suicide and the Victorian Asylum: Attempted Self-Murder in the Age of Non Restraint', *Medical History*, vol. 46, no. 2 (2002): 175–196; Sarah York, 'Alienists, Attendants and the Containment of Suicide in Public Lunatic Asylums, 1845–1890', *Social History of Medicine*, vol. 25 no. 2 (2012): 324–42.

[86] The Triennial Report on the Lunatic Asylums in the United Provinces for the Years 1909, 1910, and 1911, NAI.

adaptable but they also used these institutions for their benefit and survival. Inmates survived by forging new bonds and taking on new roles. Ross, the Superintendent in Charge of the Delhi asylum, was of the view that 'there were some very good performers on musical instruments. Hardeo Das, discharged cured, played the sitar very well indeed; and Pahulwan, Ruguath, Harphul, Ingo—all musicians. A good deal of music and card-playing goes on when the lunatics get together in the evening.'[87]

The Civil Surgeon of the Jubbulpore asylum pointed out that 'there are male attendants for male patients only. The female patients are too low to require a special attendant, one of them being a harmless monomaniac is proud and happy at this office devolving upon her, and she does it very well. I have authority to entertain female attendants should they be required at any time.'[88] Dr Fairweather of the Delhi asylum wrote, 'Ashraff Khan, the criminal lunatic ... has been gradually restored to liberty and now he goes about free and unrestrained among the other lunatics. He has even within the last few weeks been made to consider himself a kind of assistant-keeper, and has helped order among the lunatics.'[89] By acting as cook or gardener, keeper or attendant, patients not only carved a niche for themselves in these alienating institutions but tapped some status and power for themselves. Thus, there were multiple layers of power dialectics within the asylum walls, including assertion of agency and the lack thereof on the part of the inmates, whereby the logic of colonial dominance was often turned upside down.

Life in the asylum was based upon stratergies of adaptation, survival, and resistance. Resistance was sometimes subtle but incidents of 'bloody' violence were not uncommon. This violence may be ignored as the wild fury of the 'madman' or else invested with deeper meaningns, reflecting aspirations and frustrations of those deemed as 'insane'. J. B. Scriven, the Superintendent in Charge of the Lahore Lunatic Asylum, described a

[87] The Annual Report on the Lunatic Asylums in the Punjab for the Year 1883, NAI.

[88] Sir James Clark's Enquiry.

[89] The Annual Report on the Lunatic Asylums of the Punjab for the Year 1876, NAI.

violent event that occurred in the year 1870, which might be quoted at some length:

> I regret also to have to record a disastrous out-break, attended with loss of life, and severe injuries to several of the attendants, that took place in the Asylum on the 24th of March. An inmate of the Asylum named Keetapai, a non-criminal lunatic who had been under treatment for the past five years. This man is perfectly sane in all points except one, viz., his own excessive rank and importance; he considers that he is an incarnation of the deity ... as a rule he may be said to have a kind disposition, as evinced in his attention to the sick—and his great boast was that he had cured some of the patients after they had been given up by the Native Doctor and myself—and also in his love for animals. I had permitted this man to keep a dog; unfortunately a litter of pups were born, and on their growing up they became such a nuisance that I was obliged to order their being disposed [of]; this was an offence not to be forgiven, and after evidently brooding over it, he persuaded a lunatic named Guggur Sing to join him in attacking the keepers. Keetapai was heard to say, 'Oh we are lunatics, we can do what we like and kill them all, and nothing will be done to us.' Unfortunately chance favored their design. A Bhistee of the Asylum, contrary to the strictest orders, having brought two large bamboos into his house, these were intended for the sides of a Charpoy; but they proved formidable weapons in the hand of a lunatic. Keetapai, though confined in the criminal ward, was allowed to walk and sit in the garden, and under this excuse obtained possession of the bamboos, which he managed to secrete away unobserved into the Criminal ward; he immediately gave one of them to Guggur Sing, and they simultaneously attacked the Warder at the Criminal gate, knocked him down, and rushed into the garden, attacking every keeper that attempted to oppose them; unfortunately there was a lunatic named Phummon working with a 'phowrah' in the garden, who suddenly became excited by the out-break and joined in the attack; but the other lunatics took no part except some by shouting and making a noise, while others attempted to save the keepers. The first keeper they met was killed near the entrance of the Criminal ward by a fearful blow on the head, they then rushed towards the outer gate, when they were met by another Burkundaz, who they also killed. On hearing the disturbance, Mr. Wilson, the Deputy Superintendent, who was in his house, rushed into the Asylum to see what was the matter; they met him at the gate, and he received some severe blows on the head, but was eventually rescued by the servants and one of the lunatics. Phummon

and Guggur escaped from the Asylum, but were soon re-captured. On hearing of the catastrophy, I proceeded at once to the Asylum; the Police had assembled in force; the excited and violent lunatics were at once confined in the cells and order restored. By order of the Commissioner, the ringleaders, Keetapai, Guggur Sing, and Phummon were transferred to the Central Jail for greater security. A strict investigation took place, and Keetapai, Guggur Sing, and Phummon were tried for murder; but acquitted on the grounds of insanity, and ordered to be kept in confinement during Her Majesty's pleasure. This is one of those unfortunate occurrences that all Lunatic Asylums are exposed to, notwithstanding the greatest precaution; the affair was so sudden and unprovoked that the keepers had no time to combine against their assailants. I can only state that it is the first and only out-break of a serious character that has ever taken place in the Asylum since it has been under my charge (a period of 15 years), and that the utmost vigilance and precautions are taken to prevent the possibility of a recurrence.[90]

This was a day when their world was turned upside down. Three lunatics came together and participated directly in the mayhem, while the others participated by shouting and making noises. Some helped to control the violence. Two attendants were killed and the Deputy Superintendent was injured. Keetapai had predicted that nothing would happen to them as they were lunatics and in accordance with his forecast, they were sent back to the asylum after being acquitted on grounds of insanity. Keetapai was sane enough to seek vengence. The other two lunatics who participated must have felt the brunt of living behind the closed walls of the asylum.

Time and again the insane attacked the warders, and at other times, also assaulted their fellow inmates. C. C. Manifold, the Inspector General of Civil Hospitals, United Provinces, noted in the Triennial Report on the Lunatic Asylum of the Punjab for the Years 1909, 1910, and 1911:

In 1911 a lunatic named Gurdin, an inmate of the asylum for the past 5 years and who had never given indication of a tendency to develop violent symptoms, slipt [sic] into a godown in February and emerged with a chopper. Meeting another lunatic drawing water Gurdin attacked

[90] The Annual Report of the Lunatic Asylums of the Punjab for the Year 1872, NAI.

him, hacked at his neck and severed his head from his body. The murder was accomplished almost instantaneously and without any noise, and until a warder noticed Gurdin standing by the headless corpse no one realized what had happened. Seeing the warder coming towards him Gurdin threatened him with the chopper, but on the former advancing Gurdin ran into Major Cochrane's garden where Major Cochrane and some guests had assembled. Major Cochrane went straight to Gurdin and while speaking soothingly to him pinned his arms to his sides and wrested the chopper from his grasp. Major Cochrane's promptitude and skill averted the imminent danger of another murderous attack. The recognition by the Lieutenant-Governor of his prompt and courageous action was conveyed to Major Cochrane and his conduct was brought by Government to the notice of the Director-General of the Indian Medical Service. The warder, Baldeo, was rewarded with a gratuity of two months' pay. Since this case the choppers formerly used for cutting up vegetables have been replaced by other more suitable appliances thus reducing the risk of such an occurrence to a minimum.[91]

These extraordinary moments were part of the everyday existence in asylums as murder and violence were not uncommon. Lunatics were aware of the immunity they had because of their 'insanity'. These events can be regarded as the temporary fury of the insane or may be understood as few sane moments of vengeance.

***

The 'everyday' lives of the inmates revolved around work, diet, and amusement. It comprised multiple adaptations and atonements, discernments and detachments, survival and subversion at the levels of both the staff and the patients. The quotidian tales of the people and the institutions that they inhabited are quintessential when writing the social histories of madness. Alf Ludke has fervently argued that 'historical analysis of everyday permits interrogation of struggles and occasional burst out of the anonymous/nameless masses'.[92] Goffman's concept of 'underlife' has

---

[91] The Triennial Report on the Lunatic Asylum of the Punjab for the Years 1909, 1910, and 1911, National Medical Library.

[92] Alf Ludke, *The History of Everyday Life: Reconstructing Historical Experiences and Ways of Life* (Princeton: Princeton University Press, 1995), 3–4.

been used here to undermine his larger argument about asylums as 'total institutions'.[93]

This chapter argued that the lunatic asylums in colonial India were not total institutions. Neither was the isolation imposed complete nor was the discipline exercised total. The authorities realized the limits of the mentally ill, and at no point of time were all the patients confined within the asylum forced to work. Only the number of patients who were regarded as 'curables' were employed. There was a belief that employment would make the patients self-reliant and bridge the gap between the outside and inside worlds. Nevertheless, the workhouse-like nature of the asylums can be discerned as exigencies imposed by colonialism. The asylum walls were more porous than they have been imagined to be. Patients were allowed to maintain contact with their families and the families were encouraged to be responsible for them. Local communities participated in asylum activities while the patients were permitted to take rides outside the hospital. Diet and recreation can be regarded as fulcrums around which the social and the cultural lives of the patients revolved.

[93] Goffman elaborated his concept of the total institutions in his work *Asylums*, 15–22. The idea was later used and developed further by Michel Foucault in *Discipline and Punish: The Birth of the Prison*, translated by Alan Sherdian (New York: Vintage Books, 1977).

4   Case Notes and Histories

Insanity, Institutions, and Individuals

Case notes provide us with rare insights into the ways in which case histories were constructed.[1] The symptoms of insanity were documented in Indian asylums in some form or the other from the beginning of the nineteenth century onwards. These recorded histories are available in a range of sources, which include case registers, annual reports, official files, journal articles, and monographs written by the Superintendents of the mental hospitals (see Figure 4.1). This

---

[1] The case registers belonging to the mental hospitals have largely been lost. They were supposed to be a part of the institutional archives, which meant that the records had to be kept and maintained in the same institution for internal use. Since institutions such as mental hospitals gave little attention to the preservation of records of their former patients, most of the case registers have been lost. These records were never shifted to the provincial archives or the National

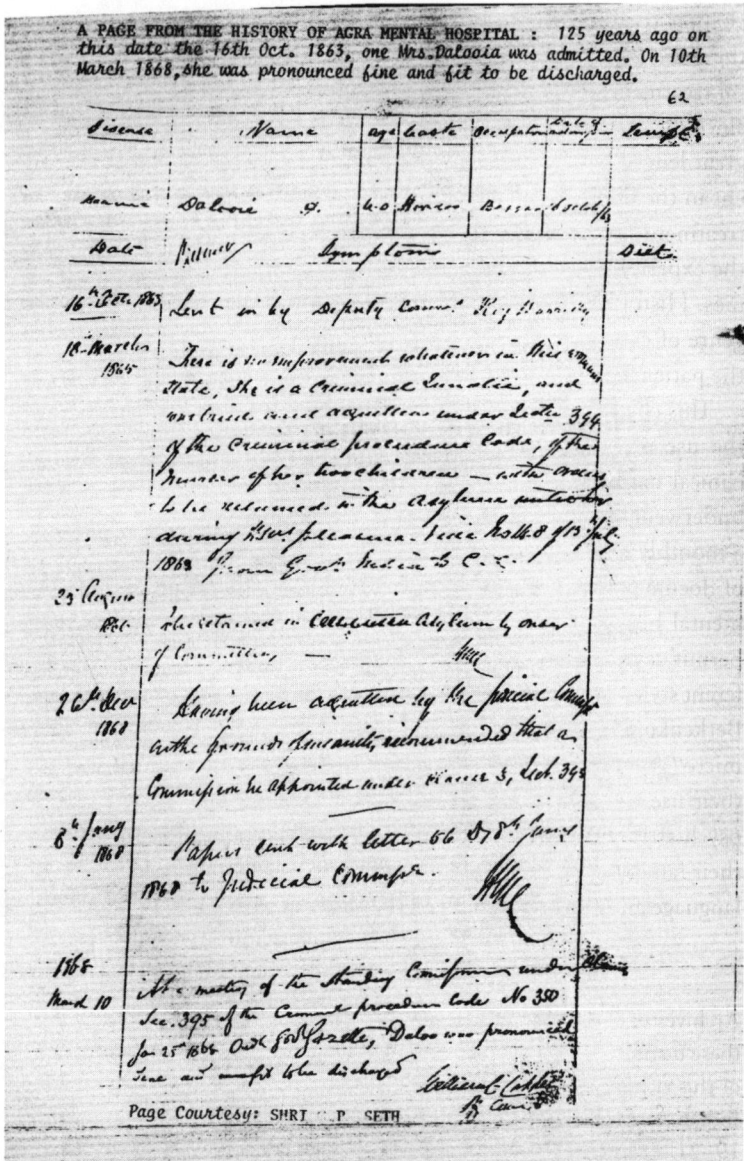

Figure 4.1 Facsimile reprint of a page from the case register of the Agra Lunatic Asylum, dated 1863–8

Source: Souvenir of 10th Annual Conference, Indian Psychiatric Society, 15–16 October 1988.

chapter tries to cull from these sources the case histories of some of the patients in order to throw light on a 'welter of insights into medical treatment and practice.'[2] The annual reports prove to be illustrative since the cases that were considered important were discussed there at great length by the Superintendents in Charge. The prejudices inherent in the documents help comprehend the notions that coloured the treatment methods. These sources also facilitate the reconstruction of the experiences of patients in the absence of their individual testimonies. Historians working on Indian asylums have largely ignored the genre of case histories since it is difficult to access clinical histories of the patients.

This chapter will attempt to understand the genre of 'case notes' and the use of language in formulating the psychiatric discourse. These clinical narratives had multiple voices inherent in them. The patients underwent monthly check-ups and the records were thus updated on a monthly basis. These monthly updates reflect the haphazard manner of documenting. The notes were written by the subordinate staff of the mental hospitals who had little education. Variations in handwriting permit us to follow changes from one medical 'scribe' to another. The different styles and handwritings also led to changes in the vocabulary. Carol Berkenkotter has highlighted the significance of macro (whole text) and micro (grammatical, lexical) techniques in her study of case histories and their use in psychiatry.[3] The language of 'madness' had a predominant psychiatric discourse hidden in it, in which there were voices of patients, their families, and the doctor. All of these were combined in a 'scientific' language and from this emerged the case notes.

Archives of India. The lack of concern of policy makers and the keepers of these institutions towards these records has been the main reason for the loss of this rich archival heritage. For details, see Shilpi Rajpal, 'Experiencing the Indian Archives', *Economic and Political Weekly*, vol. 47, no. 16 (April 2012): 19–21.

[2] Jonathan Andrews, 'Case Notes, Case Histories, and the Patient's Experience of Insanity at Gartnavel Royal Asylum, Glasgow', in the Nineteenth Century', *Social History of Medicine*, vol. 11, no. 2 (1998): 255.

[3] Carol Berkenkotter, *Patient Tales: Case Histories and the Uses of Narrative in Psychiatry* (Columbia: The University of South Carolina Press, 2008), 9.

Women, Wives, and Mothers

Scholars working on the history of psychiatry have shown that there exists a gendered history of psychiatry. Women were more commonly confined in the asylums as it was believed that women were physiologically more susceptible to insanity than men. It was also argued that their weak minds and frail bodies were not capable of handling the burdens of civilization. Elaine Showalter looking at 'two hundred years of English psychiatry' has drawn attention to the increasing number of women in asylums (through the use of census data). She writes, 'According to the census of 1871, there were 1,182 female lunatics for every 1,000 male lunatics, and 1,242 female pauper lunatics for every 1,000 male pauper lunatics. By 1872, out of 58,640 certified lunatics in England and Wales, 31,822 were women.'[4] Her work has tried to establish that not only statistically but also culturally and socially madness was a 'female malady'. However, in colonial India, men outnumbered women in the asylums. Historians working on the Indian subcontinent have shown that the ratio of men to women confined in the asylums ranged from 5:1 to 2:1.[5] This statistical evidence has allowed the questioning of the dominant view that madness was essentially a female malady. Scholars, nevertheless, agree that annual reports, case notes, and accounts of doctors reflect gendered notions of female insanity.

Waltraud Ernst suggests,

The figures indicate that in almost all the institutions designated for the admission of Indians, male patients quite clearly outnumbered female patients. In numerical terms, therefore, the situation in India in regard to

[4] Elaine Showalter, *The Female Malady: Women, Madness and English Culture, 1830–1980* (London, Virago Press, 1987), 52.

[5] Waltraud Ernst, 'Feminising Madness—Feminising the Orient: Gender, Madness and Colonialism, c. 1860–1940', in *Exploring Gender: Colonial and Post-colonial India*, edited by S. Kak and B. Pati (New Delhi: Nehru Memorial and Museum Library, 2005), 57–92; Debjani Das, 'Is Insanity a "Female Malady"? Lunatic Women in the Asylums of Bengal in the Nineteenth Century', *Social Scientist*, vol. 39, nos 5–6 (May–June 2011): 23–47. For more details, see Debjani Das, *Houses of Madness: Insanity and Asylums of Bengal in Nineteenth-Century India* (New Delhi: Oxford University Press, 2015).

sex-specific institutionalisation rates, is reversed to the one that prevailed in Britain, where women are supposed to have had a greater chance than men of finding themselves inside a mental institution.[6]

Debjani Das examines the question of female insanity in relation to the asylums of Bengal. Her study shows,

> The number of women as compared to men was 1 to 3 or 4. Based on these records reflecting on the proportion of the sexes, the superintendent surgeon stated that insanity in reality was more frequent amongst males than amongst females of the country. Even after four decades, the condition was almost similar; women constituted 21.5 per cent of the admissions in the asylums of Bengal by 1871, against 23.6 of 1870 and 20.8 of the five preceding years.[7]

C. M. Smith, the Superintendent of the Lahore asylum, observed in this context that 'on the 1st of January, 1868, there were 205 patients under treatment, viz., males 166, females 39'.[8] D. O'C. Raye, the Inspector General of Civil Hospitals, Punjab, remarked that 'on the 1st January 1895, 236 inmates remained from the previous year, of whom 187 were males and 49 females. Seventy admissions took place during the year, of these 58 were men and 12 were women'.[9] R. Heard, Inspector General of Civil Hospitals, Punjab, pointed out that 'at the commencement of the year 1922 there were 846 patients (670 males and 176 females)'.[10] A similar pattern of the male/female ratio existed in the asylums of the United Provinces. The Report on Dispensaries and Lunatic Asylums in the Province of Oudh for the Year 1869 noted that 'the patients remaining on the 31st December 1868 were male, 98 and females 42'.[11]

[6] Ernst, 'Feminising Madness', 61.

[7] Das, 'Is Insanity a "Female Malady"?': 39.

[8] The Annual Report of the Lunatic Asylums of the Punjab for the Year 1868.

[9] The Annual Report of the Lunatic Asylums of the Punjab for the Year 1895.

[10] The Annual Report on the Working of Punjab Mental Hospital for the Year 1922.

[11] The Report on Dispensaries and Lunatic Asylum in the Province of Oudh for the Year 1869.

The statistical table of the United Provinces for the year of 1904 enumerated a total population of 1,150, of which there were 881 men and 269 women.[12]

As mentioned earlier the general ratio of male to females in the asylums ranged from 5:1 to 2:1. Historians have attributed the wide gap that existed between male and female rates of confinement to the highly gendered socio-cultural conditions that were present in the Indian subcontinent. Ernst has argued that since most of the admissions in the asylums consisted 'mainly of people sent in by the police, via the magistrates, rather than those admitted by relatives seeking care and medical treatment for their beloved ones',[13] and the fact that women mostly were confined within the four walls of their houses, they were 'less likely to draw adverse attention from colonial officials authorized to send those to specialized institutions who were seen to disturb the peace and order of public places and European enclaves'.[14] Das has pointed out,

> Women who were admitted into the 'native' asylums of Bengal mainly included beggars, coolies, cultivators, labourers, fisherwomen, housewives and prostitutes, and by 1870s there were also references of insane women who prior to their admission worked as domestic servants, washerwomen, shopkeepers, and weavers. Of the different kinds of women admitted in the European Lunatic Asylum, European soldiers' wives and daughters were predominant.[15]

In the asylums of the Punjab and the United Provinces, there were several beggars, servants, labourers, farmers, prostitutes, and spinners. Wives of Europeans and Eurasians were often sent to the asylum. One rarely comes across cases of Indians voluntarily seeking admission for their wives, mothers, or daughters.

The wide gap in the male and female ratio of inmates surprised the colonial officials time and again. Charles J. Lodge Patch, the Superintendent

---

[12] Report and Returns of the Lunatic Asylums in the United Provinces for the Year 1904.

[13] Ernst, 'Feminising Madness', 62.

[14] Ernst, 'Feminising Madness', 62.

[15] Das, 'Is Insanity a "Female Malady"?': 24.

of the Lahore asylum, reproduced some of the arguments put forth by the retired Superintendent of the asylum on the issue:

In 1908, Ewens correctly ascribes this small proportion of female admissions to prejudice on the part of Indian husbands, 'notwithstanding the great advantages which may be expected from hospital treatment.' And in 1911, on the same subject, he observes 'it is very rare for a better class Indian woman to be admitted; a few who were too troublesome to be kept at home are brought to the asylum as a last resource, but the very great majority are wanderers who are picked up by the police many miles away from their homes ... There are many females who have been in the Asylum for years, about whom nothing is known not even in their names!'[16]

Patch added his own insight to his superior's view:

As it was twenty years ago, so it [is] to-day. The number of both sexes has considerably increased, but the proportions remain more or less the same. For some time past, Indian women have been forsaking the *boorkha* (veil) and the purdah system to a greater extent each year; but fathers and husbands are still filled with traditional prejudices against modern ways and modern methods of treatment. This is, perhaps, only to be expected in a country in which ninety per cent of the inhabitants are uneducated and illiterate.[17]

These arguments provide an insight into the official mindset. These officials blamed Indian traditions, customs, and social arrangements. These opinions were not completely unjustified as it was more or less considered a taboo to send womenfolk to these alien institutions. Women who were found loitering without any explanation were picked up by the police officers and were sent to the asylums. The larger problem with these arguments is their derogatory racial and gender undertones.

[16] George Francis Williams Ewens was the first Superintendent in Charge of the central Punjab Lunatic Asylum at Lahore from 1900 up till his death in 1913. Before assuming the role of the superintendent, Ewens was in charge of several jails in the Punjab. Ewens's statement is cited by Charles J. Lodge Patch, *A Critical Review of the Punjab Mental Hospitals from 1840–1930* (Lahore Record Office: Punjab Government, 1931), 81.

[17] Patch, *A Critical Review of the Punjab Mental Hospitals*, 81–2.

There exists a general consensus among historians that madness in women was ascribed to their basic biological difference. The hierarchical gradation in India was just not about the sexual difference between men and women as the pecking order was also based on the so-called civilizational difference. Patch quoted another retired Superintendent's viewpoint:

> Milne attributes the small proportion of women in the Indian Psychiatric institutions to the facts that they are not addicted to intoxicating drugs, and the process of child-birth are easier than in more civilized races. The first of his assertion is certainly true. Possibly also the second, especially in 1905 when the European woman's pelvis and abdominal organs were compressed as mechanical contraptions. If she were to be in the fashion it was extremely important that she should present to the world the wasp like waist which was then regarded as the main criterion of elegance.[18]

The civilizational difference was considered to be an important factor as far as the understanding of insanity was concerned. It was reiterated that insanity was the disease of the civilized and the 'savages' are less prone to be mentally ill since civilization induces burdens on the brain; the lesser civilized races lived simply and were thus less likely to suffer from insanity.

Hilary Marland has extensively researched on insanity and childbirth during the Victorian period. She argues that 'by the early nineteenth century an entire battery of diseases and disorders associated with reproduction was elaborated on, and puerperal insanity would fit neatly into this context as a link was "forged" between obstetrics, gynaecology and psychiatry.'[19] Marland's work focuses on the birth of puerperal insanity. The following case history from the Punjab asylum reflects the use of the category related to childbirth and insanity:

> K. 6-5-00 Section 302. Acquitted on ground of insanity. While insane through 'grief' at absence of husband killed her two children aged 3 years and 3 months, respectively by cutting their abdomen open with a rambi.

---

[18] Captain J. C. Robertson Milne was the officiating Superintendent in Charge of the Lahore Asylum from January to June 1906. His statement was cited by Patch in *A Critical Review of the Punjab Mental Hospitals*, 81.

[19] Hilary Marland, *Dangerous Motherhood: Insanity and Childbirth in Victorian Britain* (Basingstoke and New York: Palgrave Macmillan, 2004), 20.

Admitted with melancholia from which she subsequently recovered; still in asylum and sane; very rough and even cruel with other women; dull and stupid.[20]

The notion that puerperal insanity was uncommon in India was widely prevalent among psychiatrists. Das has argued that there exist few references to puerperal mania in the asylums of Bengal. She pointed out that 'according to the medical officers, it was more frequent among women in the European Asylums than among women of the "native" asylums.'[21] Certain categories of psychiatric diseases were believed not to be prevalent in India. This denial on the part of colonial officials can be attributed to their understanding related to civilizational and racial differences. However, the links between insanity and childbirth were commonly made. G. F. W. Ewens, the Superintendent of the Punjab Mental Hospital remarked:

> Indeed, in all varieties of insanity occurring at the time of childbirth there is a peculiar danger in this respect, and no child should be left with a mother unwatched under these circumstances, the mothers frequently, indeed almost always, having a strong dislike to it, and to her husband, or having delusions that may cause her to murder it.[22]

The lunatic asylums of the Punjab and the United Provinces had few cases ascribed to women suffering from insanity related to childbirth. The Triennial Report of the United Provinces for the Years 1921, 1922, and 1923 shows that 'there were 20, 23 and 24 cases respectively related to parturition and lactation'.[23] The general registers of Lahore Mental Hospital have two interesting cases describing insanity due to childbirth.

> Jumna Devi W/O Chander Lal—Date of Admission—9.12.1937—30—Housewife—C/O Dr Jagan Nath, Chaman Lain Road, Lahore—In relation to child birth—M.C. Lahore, Pauper.

[20] G. F. W. Ewens, *Insanity in India: Its Symptoms and Diagnosis: With Reference to the Relation of Crime and Insanity* (Calcutta: Thacker, Spink & co., 1908, reprint, Memphis: General Books, 2009), 227.

[21] Das, 'Is Insanity a "*Female Malady*"?': 29.

[22] Ewens, *Insanity in India*, 198.

[23] The Triennial Report on the Lunatic Asylums in the United Provinces of Agra and Oudh for the Years 1921, 1922, and 1923, NAI.

Raj Dulari W/O Chaudhary Inder Singh Midha—32—Date of Admission—5.6.1944—Hindu—Toba Tek Singh, Lyallpur—Received from Lahore—Puerperal insanity—Bill by Account.[24]

Childbirth was regarded to be a painful and frightening time in the lives of women. During the colonial period a whole set of notions regarding 'scientific motherhood' was devised. In case of Jumna Devi, she was supposedly under the care of Dr Jagan Nath who might have referred her to the mental hospital. The notes are incomplete and one cannot know the actual reasons of her insanity. It is alleged that her insanity was in relation to childbirth. The reasons could vary as she might have not been able to give birth to a male child and familial pressure would have driven her insane. Indian society was extremely patriarchal and women's inability to give birth to a male heir could have grave consequences on her physical and mental health. The madness attributable to Jumna Devi or Dulari, who allegedly suffered from puerperal insanity, may have been due to their inability to take care of her children according to the established norms of the time. Lastly, it could have been because of what is known today as postnatal depression. Therefore, the category of puerperal insanity needs to be contextualized in accordance with the Indian milieu. Insanity, after all, is a disease caused due to biological, cultural, and social factors. The social history of psychiatry should take cognizance of insanity caused due to 'the burdens of motherhood'[25] that were enforced upon women by patriarchal societies.

[24] Case Entry Register, Lahore Mental Hospital, 1944.

[25] For a discussion on this subject, see Jasodhara Bagchi, 'Representing Nationalism: Ideology of Motherhood in Colonial Bengal', *Economic and Political Weekly*, vol. 25, no. 42/43 (1990): WS65–WS71; Katherine Mayo, *Mother India*, edited and with an introduction by Mrinalini Sinha (Ann Arbor: University of Michigan Press, 2000, 1998); Tanika Sarkar, *Hindu Wife, Hindu Nation: Community, Religion and Cultural Nationalism* (Delhi: Permanent Black, 2001); Sugata Bose, *The Nation as Mother and Other Visions of Nationhood* (Gurgaon, Haryana: Penguin Viking, 2017); and Ranjana Saha, 'Modern Maternities: Discourses on Breastfeeding and Child Development in Colonial Bengal', unpublished PhD thesis, University of Delhi, 2017. In the European context, see Lynda Roper, *Oedipus & the Devil: Witchcraft, Sexuality and Religion in Early Modern Europe* (London: Routledge, 1994).

Female infanticide was widely prevalent in India due to the prefer-
ence given to the male child.[26] Some criminal cases related to women's
incarceration in the asylums were linked to the practice of infanticide.
Let us examine some of these:

M. S. T., age 30. Admitted 30.8.03. Class I. Section 302. Chronic
Melancholia. This woman killed her own child and kept the body on the
lap for 3 days until discovered. She has always been in the asylum in the
condition of melancholia, weeping and bewailing, with delusions of her
husband and 4 sons being confined close by, quite unreasonable.[27]
[...] Mst. D. 25-07-97 Aquitted on ground of insanity. Killed her child
by throwing it on the ground when in state of melancholia—noticed in
Asylum to be very cruel to children. Has not recovered.[28]

The sex and age of the child murdered is unclear in these case histories.
The socio-economic processes have to be contextualized in order to comprehend the practices of infanticide, and it should be kept in mind that
the mother's decision to kill her child (especially female) could have been
the result of pressure generated by immediate family. Puerperal insanity
in India was not simply related to mania or melancholia. Insanity and
childbirth in India had a latent connection to infanticide. This connection cannot be delved into in detail due to a serious paucity of sources. If
infanticide was peculiar to the Indian milieu then puerperal insanity was
a typical disease of Victorian England. Its use in the Indian asylum was
a result of the colonial transference of medical ideas.

Puerperal insanity was not the only category that mirrored the
intimate linkages between the woman and her physiology. Women's

[26] For further readings on female infanticide, see L. S. Vishwanath,
'Efforts of Colonial State to Suppress Female Infanticide: Use of Sacred Texts,
Generation of Knowledge', *Economic and Political Weekly*, vol. 33, no. 19 (May
1998): 1104–12; Satadru Sen, 'The Savage Family: Colonialism and Female
Infanticide in Nineteenth Century India', *Journal of Women's History*, vol. 14,
no. 3 (2002): 53–79; Anshu Malhotra, *Gender, Caste and Religious Identities:
Restructuring Class in Colonial Punjab* (New Delhi: Oxford University Press,
2002), among others.

[27] Ewens, *Insanity in India*, 219.

[28] Ewens, *Insanity in India*, 225.

biological processes were integrated into the symptomology of insanity. Her menstruation's cyclic rhythms were considered markers of her sanity/insanity. Overbeck-Wright, the Superintendent of the Agra asylum, remarked:

> During menstruation women are much more liable to suffer from insanity and various neuroses. An enquiry among female criminals in Europe elicited the fact that in a very large percentage indeed the crime was perpetrated during a menstrual period. Most cases, too, of kleptomania and other impulsive insanities among women occur during the process of menstruation. In asylums, in the female sections, maniacs are always more maniacal, melancholics more depressed during a menstrual period. This point is well worth remembering, as it has important medico-legal bearings.[29]

Das has aptly pointed out that 'the irregular flow of menstrual cycle was considered as one of the most important causes of women's insanity. The medical officers often regarded a woman as sane when she had her menstrual flow regularly and a woman as insane when she got irregular menses'.[30] Yannick Ripa has looked at incarceration of women diagnosed with insanity in nineteenth-century France, and she has argued that 'the normalisation of femininity involved a healthy menstrual cycle. When the patient arrived in the asylums the doctors would observe her periods and take note of regularity, quantity and colour of the blood'.[31] Thomas Laqueur's path-breaking work has demonstrated how by the beginning of the nineteenth century, differences between the sexes were established in oppositional terms.[32] This clearly had deep sociocultural implications. Marland has argued that the invention of puerperal insanity 'led to the office of the midwife to be taken over by male practitioners, who offered protection in return for recognition of their expertise to

---

[29] Alexander William Overbeck-Wright, *Lunacy in India* (London: Bailliere, Tindall & Cox, 1921), 352.

[30] Das, 'Is Insanity a "*Female Malady*"?': 34.

[31] Yannick Ripa, *Women and Madness: The Incarceration of Women in Nineteenth Century France* (Cambridge: Polity Press, 1990), 139.

[32] Thomas Laqueur, *Making Sex: Body and Gender from the Greeks to Freud* (Cambridge: Harvard University Press, 1990), 5.

monitor and take action against the dangers of childbearing'.[33] She further argued that the link forged between obstetrics and psychiatry led to the redefining of women's proper role and functions.[34] The categories from hysteria to neurasthenia and from delusions to grief became synonymous with women's weak intellect, menstruating cycles, and feeble bodies. The case histories mentioned in Overbeck-Wright's monograph would help in elucidating the point further.

> At the present moment, in Agra asylum there is a patient suffering from a delusion that her husband (who was really a farrier in a British cavalry regiment) was a most influential and important personage, knighted by King Edward's own hands; that he was rich and well-to-do, but foully murdered in South Africa shortly after the war. (He really went out there with the Imperial Yeomanry, and stayed there after peace was declared, deserting his wife). Since then, she states, the Roman Catholics have formed a conspiracy to 'obtain possession of her accumulation and children,' and prevent her marrying 'her sole guardian and protector, to whom she became legally engaged in a Magistrate's Court on a certain date' (her 'sole legal guardian and protector,' as a matter of fact, being the superintendent of goal where she was kept as an under-trail prisoner, and already married). Delusions may be transitory and of but little import [importance] as in practically every case of mania. It is only when permanent or fixed that they have vital bearing on the case.[35]

One can cite another case:

> At the present moment in the Agra asylum there is a woman who murdered her child under such conditions. She has been well-to-do, but her husband died and adversity came on her way. She was living with some distant relatives, along with her daughter. At night the mother and child occupied one room. She was worried about money and about her daughter's future and gradually felt the desire come upon her to kill the child, the only being in the world she had to love and to love her. Again and again she implored those with whom she was living to separate them, to keep them apart and gave them her reasons. They simply scoffed, and to

[33] Marland, *Dangerous Motherhood*, 7.
[34] Marland, *Dangerous Motherhood*, 15.
[35] Overbeck-Wright, *Lunacy in India*, 11.

emphasize their incredulity took to locking in the mother and child at night, and the thing the women dreaded and fought against came to pass. She was tried and sent to asylum under Section 47I, C.P.C. Here the permanent and underlying wish of the person was the safety and welfare of her child, as evidenced by her efforts to remove it from the danger and keep temptations out of her way. The immediate desire, *the obsession*, under certain conditions—her being left alone with her child—impelled her to the deed from which her whole being revolted and her every action, when removed from these conditions, was antagonistic.[36]

In the first case, the woman's delusions were supposed to have resulted from her feeble mind. Her inability to deal with reality paved the way to her delusions of grandeur about her husband and life. In the second case, the woman's grief was the result of her overt emotions. Both the narratives constructed by the Superintendent in Charge reflect his sympathies but also mirror gendered biased notions. They show how feeble mind and overt emotions were inextricably linked to women's biology. What was thoroughly being sidelined is their displacement and social factors such as the insecurities of widows and unwed women in a patriarchal set-up that was innate and left them in an unsettled state of mind.

Das has argued,

In Bengal, the issue of puerperal mania did not limit itself to the question of maintaining or breaking the norms of femininity. Instead it pointed to a more complicated medical issue. It raised certain questions about the treatment of women's illnesses: for instance, what led to so many cases of puerperal mania or fever? Was it related to hygiene? Did women give birth in unhygienic conditions? Therefore, this particular cause of women's insanity questions both her reproductive and mental health.[37]

Das underplays the question of femininity which was intrinsically tied to women's position. As she sees it, her position in turn was responsible in deciding what sort of medical, social, and economic facilities would be provided to her. Her mental health was impaired by the stifled milieu in which she was forced to live. Insanity in the Indian milieu might

[36] Overbeck-Wright, *Lunacy in India*, 14.
[37] Das, 'Is Insanity a "*Female Malady*"?': 29.

not be the result of rebellion against the patriarchal norms but, on the contrary, these norms could have been an important and a deep source related to the melancholy of women. Indrani Sen has aptly argued that 'the subordinate social status and family role that is generally assigned to women in most societies—especially among poorer sections of society—can create situations of considerable stress that can be catalytic factors in the case of female mental illness.'[38]

The annual reports elucidated that a large number of women who were incarcerated were neither mothers nor wives. These women were found wandering around without any 'valid' explanation. Their supposed licentiousness would have led to their incarceration. This category included prostitutes, wanderers, and ascetic women. Mothers were usually sequestered in the asylum if they had committed infanticide. Wives of Eurasians or Europeans were more likely to be sent to the asylums than the wives of Indian gentlemen. Their confinement in asylums was determined by the overwhelming feminine definitions of the time. Whether it was the West or the East, the definition of women's madness had an intimate relation to her feminine roles. This biased categorization became a vicious circle that denied her human agency. Madness at large might not be a 'female malady' but one of the most essential maladies of women was supposed to be their 'inherent' insanity.

The 'Idiots', the Poor, and the Homeless

This section looks at groups of people who belonged to the larger category of the 'poor' such as the homeless, the 'nomads', and the 'idiots'. These people often (but not always) became permanent members of psychiatric institutions. Some sections amongst these groups were often targeted by the state, but the case histories have also shown that the poor and often the dependents (who were discarded by their families) used these institutions as a 'refuge' against hard times. This is not to deny the coercive side of psychiatric power that led to the criminalization of such itinerant ways of life.

---

[38] Indrani Sen, 'The Memsahib's "Madness": The European Woman's Mental Health in Late Nineteenth Century India', *Social Scientist*, vol. 33, nos 5–6 (May–June 2005): 27.

One particular group that benefitted from these institutions was that of the 'idiots' or 'imbeciles', or 'mentally retarded' as they are known, and epileptics. David Wright has worked on the Earlswood asylum for 'idiots' in England. He asserts that, "'Lunatics", by contrast, referred to all those who, thought previously "sane", suffered from a temporary or permanent impairment of mental ability. Idiots were individuals who never had mind'.[39] In the changing socio-economic times families often failed to take the responsibility of the mentally disabled, and India had no separate asylums for 'idiots'. The mentally disabled were often abandoned by their families. A noteworthy case of the so called wolf-child,[40] sheds light on the ways these abandoned children were treated in the lunatic asylums.

> One of the epileptics has an interesting history. She is a girl of about 8 years of age, and is said to have been found in the jangle by a man when ploughing his fields, and was believed by him to be a 'wolf-child'. When brought to the asylum, she was extremely timid, and tried to hide herself in corners; she would not speak, but only uttered a peculiar kind of whine. When any one went near her or spoke to her she seemed afraid of being struck, and held up her hands to defend herself. There were some scars on her arms. When food was given to her, she always smelt it before putting it to her mouth. Great pains were taken with the child to try and draw out any latent intelligence that might be in her, but repeated severe attacks of epilepsy have reduced her to even a lower state of idiotcy than she was in before.[41]

[39] David Wright, *Mental Disability in Victorian England* (New York: Oxford University Press, 2001), 10.

[40] There exists a long history of stories related to so-called feral children or 'wolf' children. The archetypal tale is that of Mowgli of *The Jungle Book* written by Rudyard Kipling. However, social scientists have questioned the existence of 'wolf children'. Some have argued that these children in actual suffered from infantile autism while others believe that these stories are nothing more than urban myths. For further readings, see Michael P. Carroll, 'The Folkloric Origin of Modern "Animal-Parented Children" Stories', *Journal of Folklore Research*, vol. 21, no. 1 (April 1984): 63–8; Deanna K. Kreisel, 'Wolf Children and Automata: Bestiality, Boredom at Home and Abroad', *Representations*, vol. 96, no. 1 (2006): 21–47.

[41] The Annual Report of the Lunatic Asylums of the Punjab for the Year 1876, NAI.

The Annual Report for the next year stated:

> The so called 'wolf-child' mentioned in the last report, and who has apparently then fallen in abject state than ever from repeated epileptic fits, soon afterwards began to improve; she was temporarily at least cured of her epilepsy, and with returning health she became lively and playful. She came to understand some things that were said to her, but never attempted to speak. She was transferred to Secundra Orphanage, Agra, in June last, the principal of that institution having kindly offered to take charge of her. In reply to recent inquiries regarding her, I was informed that she has had no return of the epileptic fits, that she enjoys a game at ball with lady in charge, but does not talk to other children in the institution. The pleasure she takes in the play is stated to be the only gleam of intelligence she has given.[42]

It is not clear whether the girl was mentally disabled or was just an epileptic. She whined and hid away since she was abandoned as an infant and had lived a secluded life in the jungle. The girl was in a state of reticence due to lack of sociability. Abandoned children and neglected family members certainly derived benefit from these institutions. Epileptics and 'idiots' formed an important category in the lunatic asylums. Sometimes they were 'transferred to the poor houses or orphanages as a more appropriate place for their detention'[43] but they often spent a large part of their lives in these mental institutions. The 'benevolent' colonial state demonstrated its philanthropic nature by providing 'the gleam of intelligence' to 'native epileptics'.

Some religious practices were regarded as the cause of insanity among 'natives'. One group that often (not always) appears in the annual reports of the asylum is that of faqirs. Hindu and Muslim religious and healing practices were condemned and religion itself was often linked to insanity. Dr Wise, the Superintendent in Charge at the Dacca asylum, wrote, 'Religious exaltation or excitement is far from being uncommon. It occurs generally among Mohammedans faqueers, mullahs or public

---

[42] The Annual Report of the Lunatic Asylums of the Punjab for the Year 1877, NAI.

[43] The Annual Report of the Lunatic Asylums of the Punjab for the Year 1878, NAI.

readers in mosques. Among Hindoos it is unknown ... It is not likely
that among a race so careless of the present, and without any anxieties
for the future, that religious insanity in any form should be found'.[44]
The language used is racialized and communalized, which reflects the
ways in which Indian religious and cultural practices were belittled. A
large number of wandering beggars, religious mendicants, and faqirs
were locked up in asylums. The following case is an interesting example
that illustrates how faqirs were looked upon with suspicion and were
frequently deemed as 'insane':

> It appears that on the night of the 5th August 1855, the prosecutor tied
> 12 annas in a handkerchief and put the handkerchief under his pillow
> and went to sleep. On getting up next morning he found that his handker-
> chief and the money in it had been stolen during the night (apparently).
> He was searching for the Handkerchief when one Mustan Shah came
> up to him with the Handkerchief tied on his head and being asked by
> Prosecutor where he had got the handkerchief from, said one Nuthoo
> had given it to him. Prosecutor accordingly went and asked Nathoo if he
> knew anything about the matter. He was told by Nuthoo that he had not
> given the handkerchief to Mustan Shah ... There is also evidence to prove
> that Mustan Shah Fakeer was not in his right mind, when he took the
> handkerchief and the money in it, it is likewise established that Mustan
> Shah was for a long time insane before he committed the offence with
> which he is charged. The medical office states that Mustan Shah was of
> weak intellect when he was first placed under his treatment and that he
> considered that the man had been of unsound mind, a long time before
> he was examined. The medical officer also says that Mustan Shah has not
> improved since he has been under Medical treatment, and he does not
> think it probable that the man will ever recover.[45]

Mustan Shah had committed petty theft. He was not sent to jail but
rather to the medical officer who declared him insane with no hope

[44] Sir James Clark's Enquiry as to the Care and the Treatment of Lunatics,
Home Dept./Public Branch, File Nos 22–3, December 19, 1868, NAI.

[45] Mustan Shah of Nursingpoor District, Saugor Division, deemed insane.
From A. A. Roberts, Sessions Judge, Saugor and Nerbudda Territories, to
Secretary of Government, dated Jubbulpoor, 1 April 1856, North Western
Provinces, Criminal Judicial Proceedings, April 1856. (I owe this particular
reference to Professor William Pinch.)

of recovery. In a further enquiry, it was made clear that he was not a threat to public safety.[46] Mustan Shah's crime was his mendicant way of life. The relation between mendicancy and madness was based on an 'unproductive' way of life. It was criminal to the extent that a religious mendicant did not conform to the idea of utility or productivity and his 'spiritual experiences' did not conform to ideas of Western religiosity. Nile Green points out that throughout the nineteenth century religious men were linked to crime and insanity.[47] He further states that '[n]one of these holy men were considered more dubious—more superstitious and reactionary—than the dervishes and faqırs.'[48] William Pinch has analysed the role of ascetics in Indian history. He cited William Sleeman to show the perpetual distrust related to religious men. Sleeman wrote, 'There is hardly any species of crime that is not throughout India perpetrated by men in the disguise of these religious mendicants; and almost all such mendicants are really men in disguise.'[49] One can find the resonance of this distrust in the medical records as well. Ewens, the Superintendent of the Lahore Lunatic Asylum, remarked, 'When a man falls into trouble or becomes destitute (and most who recover from insanity) promptly go out into the world as faqirs, the vast majority of whom are habitual consumers of hemp in the form of *charas*, as indeed are all religious mendicants, and I have no hesitation in saying become more or less insane.'[50] Littlewood argued that 'dysphoric moods and

---

[46] Mustan Shah of Nursingpoor District, Saugor Division, deemed insane. From A. A. Roberts, Sessions Judge, Saugor and Nerbudda Territories, to Secretary of Government, dated Jubbulpoor, 1 April 1856, North Western Provinces, Criminal Judicial Proceedings, April 1856.

[47] Nile Green, 'Jack Sepoys and the Dervishes: Islam and the Indian Soldier in Princely Hyderabad', *Journal of the Royal Asiatic Society*, vol. 18, no. 1 (2008): 31–46.

[48] Green, 'Jack Sepoys and the Dervishes': 31.

[49] Sir William Sleeman, 'A Report on the System of Megpunnaism or, the Murder of Indigent Parents for their Young Children (Who Are Sold as Slaves) as It Prevails in the Delhi Territories, and the Native States of Rajpootana, Ulwar, and Bhurtpore (Serampore, 1839)', 11, cited in W. R. Pinch, *Warrior Ascetics and Indian Empires* (Cambridge: Cambridge University Press, 2006), 238.

[50] Ewens, *Insanity in India*, 4.

"unusual actions" were locally recognised in India, nor necessarily as a physical or mental illness, rather as part of totally different patterns of experience and order—as spirit possession or rituals of mourning, or as events in the course of initiation, sorcery or warfare'.[51] He further asserted that 'the colonial doctors and administrators found it difficult, given the variety of local patterns ... to fit them into restrictive categories already identified in European hospitals'.[52]

C. A. Bayly argues that 'the colonial order emerged strengthened from the ordeal of 1857 and consequently, in the wake of the Rebellion new methods of formal and informal surveillance were employed. Sufi religious orders, networks of mosque preachers, temples and monasteries became even more marginal to the British and were regarded as dangerous'.[53] Throughout the colonial period, faqirs continued to be looked upon with suspicion. The Agra case registers have a number of cases of faqirs who were incarcerated in the mental hospitals even in the twentieth century. An illustrative case is of the faqir Sadhu Jalender Nath, who spent 45 years of his life in the hospital:

Sadhu Jalender Nath—35 years—Hindu Faqir-Beggar—Admitted to the Agra Mental Hospital on 21.6.07—Dementia—Dull—Blind—no work—Died on 29.12.52 at 1.30. A.M.[54]

Sadhu Jalender Nath was 35 years old when he was admitted in the hospital in 1907 and died on 29 December 1952. He was diagnosed with age-related dementia at the age of 35. His case history is only available from the year 1946 to 1952 and the case notes are fragmentary. It was stated that he was old and blind. He did not participate in any sort

---

[51] Roland Littlewood, 'Colonialism and Psychiatry', in *Colonialism and Psychiatry*, edited by Dinesh Bhugra and Roland Littlewood (New Delhi: Oxford University Press, 2002), 2.

[52] Littlewood, 'Colonialism and Psychiatry', 2.

[53] C. A. Bayly, *Empire and Information: Intelligence Gathering and Social Communication in India, 1750–1870* (New Delhi: Cambridge University Press, 1999), 338.

[54] A short summary of the case is discussed here. The complete case history is available in Appendix no. 1, Case no. 24; Register nos 58 and 59, the Agra Mental Hospital.

of work. Words like 'infirm', 'dull', 'old', and 'senile' have been used inter-changeably. There is no discussion on his mental state in the case notes. We find that mendicants' ways of life were often targeted. William Pinch argues that 'sadhus generally were seen as a potential source of criminal mischief by officials of the Raj is evident in the publication in 1913 of a police handbook in Urdu that described the various religious orders and, in detailed line drawings, examples of representative figures down to the distinctive sandalwood-paste sect marks.'[55]

The nineteenth century led to the criminalization of the poor in the West. The implications for the colonies were much more severe as the pseudo-scientific epistemological formulations on criminology led to the criminalization of all those who did not (or could not) live a sedentary life. Nineteenth-century annual reports show that beggars, cultivators, and labourers were to be found in these institutions in large numbers. The Agra case registers show that a considerable section of vagrants lived a large part of their lives in the mental institutions.

> Rashid Hakim Khan—47—Mohamedan—Vagrant—Transferred from the Benares Mental Hospital to the Agra Metal Hospital on 5.12.42—Dementia—quiet—no work—dull—no work—confused—working in WS compound—no work—wants to go home.[56]

Rashid Hakim Khan, a 47-year-old vagrant, was transferred from the Benares Mental Hospital, which was a criminal mental hospital. This indicates that he was probably picked up by the police (like most of the vagrants) for some petty crime. After a period of short stay in the Benares Mental Hospital, he was transferred to the Agra Mental Hospital. The transfer points to the fact that he was not a typical 'criminal' insane. He was described as dull, quiet, and confused and his case notes are available from 1942 to 1947. Mr Khan continued to live in the Agra Mental Hospital even after 1947 but his case notes are not available.

---

[55] William R. Pinch, *Peasants and Monks in British India* (Berkeley; University of California Press, 1996), 8.

[56] A short summary of the case is discussed here. The complete case history is available in Appendix no. 2, Case no 54; Register no. 66, the Agra Mental Hospital, NAI.

He was diagnosed with dementia related to old age. He did not actively participate in hospital work, which would have been an impediment to his freedom. Mr Khan's case is a representative one since the Agra case registers have a number of cases of the homeless who were sent to the mental hospital. The criminalization of vagrancy has a long history in the West. In India, as vagrancy laws were still not in place, mental hospitals were used for clearing the streets.

The 'poor'—including the 'idiots', the 'epileptics', the vagrants, and all those who had mobile ways of life—lived their lives on the margins and were (and are) considered 'unproductive' or 'dangerous' or both by the state and society. The colonial state often tried to confine this miniscule section of the 'poor', who were regarded as 'dangerous'. This section was not necessarily insane but their inability to cope with socio-economic fluctuations (homelessness due to poverty), intellectual inability (mentally challenged), or the itinerant ways of life (pastoralists and other communities who travelled from one place to another for work) were regarded as reason enough for their incarceration.[57] The epistemological linkage that was forged during the period between the poor and the criminal had deeper ramifications. Meena Radhakrishna rightly argues that 'as work-shy vagrant and beggars, they join the socially homogenous category of the "poor". From here they finally re-emerge as a special type of criminal that was legislated against by the state—namely the beggar offender.'[58]

Criminals and Delinquents

Asylums provided the colonial state with a place for incarcerating 'dangerous' Indians. 'Criminal lunatics' constituted the largest category that occupied the lunatic asylums throughout the colonial period. The category was a wide one since it included murderers and also those who had committed petty crimes. It also referred to those who could

[57] The debates related to the poor, the vagrants, and the 'criminalization' of tribes have been discussed in Chapter 3.

[58] Meena Radhakrishna, 'Laws of Metamorphosis: From Nomad to Offender', in *Challenging the Rule(s) of Law: Colonialism, Criminology and Human Rights in India*, edited by Kalpana Kannabiran and Ranbir Singh (New Delhi: Sage, 2009), 4.

not be categorized in any definite group such as 'political criminals'. The 'criminal lunatic' was thus at the same time a 'definite' and an 'ambiguous' category. The word 'delinquent' has thus been used here to dismantle the umbrella category of 'criminal lunatics'. The term 'delinquent' here refers to those who were not considered to be good subjects due to their wayward behaviour. The available legal framework was used to put them behind asylum walls. This section looks at some illustrative cases belonging to the so called 'problematic' segment of society.

Michel Foucault while discussing the power of psychiatric knowledge elaborates on the process by which the psychiatrist becomes a doctor-judge. This process impinged upon the legal-judicial system. Foucault remarks,

> It is true that expert psychiatric opinion contributes nothing to knowledge, but this is not what matters. Its essential role is to legitimize, in the form of scientific knowledge, the extension of punitive power to something that is not a breach of the law. What is essential is that it makes it possible to resituate the punitive action of judicial power within a general corpus of reflected techniques for the transformation of individuals.[59]

The power was used and abused in the colonial milieu. The following examples would help in elaborating the point in detail:

A.D. 21-10-02. Theft. Class I. Unable to plead.
  Arrested for stealing a blanket valued at Rs 3–8; he had had six previous convictions for similar offences, and had undergone an aggregate of six years in jail and 78 stripes.
  'He was served with a notice of ejection under section 210, C.P.C. He paid no attention to this, and was arrested shortly after for theft, present offence'. 'A. D. is of the weak intellect, and from his demeanour in court, it is clear that he has not the slightest sense of responsibility for the offences he commits,' though otherwise harmless and seems unable when at liberty to refrain from thieving.

[59] Michel Foucault, *Abnormal: Lectures at College de France, 1974–75*, translated by Graham Burchell (London: Verso, 2003), 18.

Regarded on admission as a chronic maniac—much improved in a few months and was discharged to stand trial on 19-06-03.[60]

A. D. was sentenced to six years of jail time and 78 stripes. The crime of repetitive thefts and his 'inability' to stand trial left the authorities helpless and thus the asylums were used as a correctional facility to 'reform' such chronic offenders as him. The consciousness of crime and guilt was considered important to declare someone a criminal, and by extension, as a marker of sanity. The absence of guilt, therefore, is regarded as insanity. There is little evidence of insanity in A. D.'s case notes. The labels 'weak intellect' and 'chronic mania' have been used to describe his inability to plead. He is not 'dangerous' in a conventional way but his crime of repetition puts him in the category of an offender. Thereby, these case notes of the patient indicate that he was treated in the mental institutions as an 'offender' and not a patient. In other words, the mental hospitals were an extension and came 'from the womb' of the punitive order.[61] The case is an evocative one since it shows how identities were constructed in medical records. The following case would elucidate the point further:

> 1-5-00 Acquitted on grounds of insanity under section 454. Had been of weak intellect for some years, said to be wandering lunatic, entering bungalows and stealing articles without regard to their value or utility to himself.
> A demented chronic maniac, very destructive. Still in Asylum.[62]

This particular patient's crimes were trespassing and theft. Colonial rationality, which was deeply tied to the notion of value or utility, was not able to forgive a repeat offender who continuously breached the tight class lines. The British system used a variety of institutions such as reformatories, jails, asylums, and convict colonies to discipline these delinquents. The records of this patient attest to the fact that only those

---

[60] Ewens, *Insanity in India*, 252.

[61] Biswamoy Pati, 'Confining "Lunatics": The Cuttack Asylum, c. 1864–1906', *Society, Medicine and Politics in Colonial India*, edited by Biswamoy Pati and Mark Harrison (New York: Routledge, 2018).

[62] Ewens, *Insanity in India*, 254.

were sent to the asylums who were considered 'dangerous'. Insanity was thus constructed in order to justify the coercive action of the colonial state. This is not to argue that all the people 'lurking around' were insane, but that only those people were sent to the asylum whose assumed or real madness was considered to be a threat to the social order.

The category of 'criminal lunatic' had several layers. Patch, while discussing the absurdity of lunacy laws in India, pointed out:

> In India, as in most civilised countries, the insane individual is 'acquitted on grounds of insanity'. However, although he has been acquitted, he is still, paradoxically, classed as criminal lunatic. There are three classes of criminal lunatics in Indian mental hospitals. The first (class i) are those who have never stood their trail, because they are too insane to understand the nature of their proceedings in a court or for some other reason. Class ii are those who have been acquitted on grounds of insanity and Class iii, those in whose case a defence of insanity may never be raised. The latter have been duly sentenced for their crimes, have broken down mentally while serving their sentences in a jail and have been admitted to the mental hospital in consequence.[63]

The criminal insane formed the so-called most productive class of these mental institutions. Patch, quoting Ewens, remarked that 'without his aid, the native staff would have to be multiplied four or five times'.[64] It was the second category of criminal lunatics who performed most of the tasks at the Lahore Mental Hospital. In most cases, their utility hindered their freedom. If criminal lunatics in this class had fewer chances of gaining their freedom, patients of the third category had zero probability of attaining their freedom. A significant case of a category III patient from the Lahore Mental Hospital is as follows:

> Pahloo—26—Date of Admission—19.12.1930–post encephalitis— Muslim—cultivator—convicted of the offence of thefts of a coat with Railway badges and buttons—sentenced to eighteen months of

---

[63] Charles J. Lodge Patch, 'Birth of a Hospital', unpublished, typescript account of the mental hospital in Lahore, Private Papers, Mss Eur F544, British Library, 281–2.

[64] Patch, 'Birth of a Hospital', 280.

rigorous imprisonment including one month of solitary confinement—talks incoherently and unintelligently—dirty is his habits—behaves like a lunatic—admits his crime—memory is fair and good—does not seem to suffer from any hallucination or delusion—appears to be feeble minded—always stealing others things—a very troublesome patient—repeats over and over again that he is sane—well behaved and obedient—teases others—steals other patients things—affectionately embraces others, sodomist—desires to go home—same, masturbates—sexual pervert, tremors, flow of saliva constant, post encephalitic symptoms—gets epileptic attacks about twice a month—semi-conscious—progressive loss of weight—referred to hospital—died of general debility on 13.2.1947.

Pahloo is described as suffering from post-encephalitis.[65] Encephalitis is a viral infection affecting the brain, the causes of which are not known. There were a number of encephalitis epidemics that occurred during and after World War I. German E. Berrios has pointed out that 'during the early 1920s, encephalitis lethargica was shown to be complicated by similar behaviour; neuroleptics and other drugs have also been found to cause catatonia-like states. Reduced to a syndrome, catatonia limped along until it began to disappear in the developed countries after the 1940s; however, cases are still seen in third-world countries.'[66] He also pointed out that in cases of post-encephalitis, symptoms were similar to 'most-schizophrenic symptoms.'[67] There is no discussion of his disease in the case notes. His behaviour was his disease, which was generally regarded as the symptoms of illness and not sickness itself.

The case notes do not describe him as 'dangerous' in a conventional way. Even then he was sentenced for a longer duration along with a month of solitary imprisonment. Solitary punishment was generally given to patients who were dangerous to themselves or others. It will be difficult to fathom whether Pahloo was insane or the system drove

---

[65] A short summary of the case is discussed here. The complete case history is available in Appendix no. 10 (file and register numbers not available [found as loose papers]), the Lahore Mental Hospital.

[66] German E. Berrios, *The History of Mental Symptoms: Descriptive Psychopathology since the Nineteenth Century* (Cambridge: Cambridge University Press, 1996), 381.

[67] Berrios, *The History of Mental Symptoms*, 406.

him to the edge of his sanity. His initial case notes mentioned that he 'repeats over and over again that he is sane' and was also regarded as 'well behaved and obedient'. The terms 'unintelligent' and 'feeble-minded' describe his inability to rectify his mistakes of stealing, which was regarded as a salient feature of his illness. His alleged incompetence was regarded as his culpability. Pahloo spent the remaining years of his life in the hospital for stealing a coat and is a typical case belonging to category III of criminal lunatics. As he broke down mentally during his sentence, his alleged insanity became real in the eyes of the colonial state when he started to 'masturbate' and 'sodomise' other inmates. His chances of getting out became minimal once he was defined as a sexual pervert. 'Perversion' and 'danger', argues Foucault, were 'stitched together' and were 'the essential theoretical core of expert medico-legal opinion'.[68] He was, therefore, classed as the most dangerous among criminals. The colonial state viewed masturbation and sodomy as unpardonable sins and crimes against humanity. Nonetheless, what is worth remembering is that Pahloo was not incarcerated for sodomy or masturbation but for stealing a coat.

The psychiatric power became a correctional force that was employed on the mad and the delinquent. The following case from the Agra Mental Hospital is one of the most evocative examples:

Bachu Lal—38—Thakur—Benares Mental Hospital—NAD—committed a dacoity at a bank at Ootacamund—Sentenced to transportation for life (25 years) but the sentence was reduced to 10 years—26.1.34 arrived at Port Blair—assaulted a deputy jailor in Andaman—burnt government clothing house—left Port Blair—arrived at Naini central prison—Transferred to Benares Mental Hospital—Kicked hospital attendant—tore up bed sheets—Arrived at Agra Mental Hospital on 16.9.38—Violent and dangerous—warn staff—A sharp piece of iron was found with his possession—kicked attendant Jafail Ahmad—noisy and demonstrative threatens to go on hunger strike—sensible no work—Discharged on 21-11-38 under section 31.[69]

---

[68] Foucault, *Abnormal*, 34.

[69] A short summary of the case is discussed here. The complete case history is available in Appendix no. 3, Case no 69; Register no. 61, the Agra Mental Hospital, NAI.

The case of Bachu Lal shows the extent to which the boundaries were blurred between crime, delinquency, and insanity. The medical category of 'NAD' commonly refers to 'no abnormality detected'. This could refer to physical or mental symptoms. There is no other description of his disease. Lal's case shows repeated resistance to treatment, which was read as a marker of his insanity. He assaulted the Deputy Jailor, burned a government clothing house, kicked a Hospital Assistant, threatened to go on hunger strike, and tore bed sheets. The violence that colonialism generated provoked the colonized subjects to resist the establishment. The state regarded these forms of resistance as markers of insanity and punished the so-called deviant for fighting back. Lal fought and rose against the colonial order in every possible way. He was finally discharged after four years of punishment. The case is significant not only because he was a nuisance and the authorities failed to control his behaviour but also because his resistance paved the way to his freedom. This extraordinary case reveals that sometimes authoritarian systems did fail. It also shows that at times not only did prisoners feign insanity to escape harsh punishment but also that the state used the label of insanity to discipline or humiliate difficult prisoners. At the same time, Lal's behaviour shows the limitations of the psychiatric structure that was repeatedly unsuccessful in ascribing and correcting him with its most 'modern' tools.

Some cases elucidate the ways in which asylums were also used as a site for suppressing dissent:[70]

> Mr. H., an Irishman by birth. On most subjects he could talk in perfect sane manner; but he believed that he was a Duke of Normandy, Grand Duke of the Grant Duke of Lancaster, and a General in the British Army. His pay as a General he believed to have been appropriated by her Majesty on oranges. He was bitterly rancorous against the British Government, and had been publically made a Mussalman in the Jama Masjid here under the name of Ahmed Din, intending afterward to make his way to Kabul and offer his services to Amir; but he was arrested by police and sent to asylum. His Mussalman friends were annoyed at being thus deprived of their proselyte, and gave some trouble by their visits, and by their threats to memorialise Government on the iniquity of making a

[70] Anirudh K. Kala, Alok Sarin, and Sanjeev Jain, 'The Psychiatrist's Partition', *Himal South Asian*, vol. 20, no. 8 (August 2007): 3.

man out to be insane because he had turned Muhammadan. After a residence of two months Mr. H. was transferred to Colaba Asylum, and his departure was a relief, for on more than one occasion he managed in some way or another to send out fictitious extracts from the newspaper, which have been lent to him, giving grossly exaggerated accounts of the progress of the Russians in Central Asia, and calling upon all Mussalmans to aid them on their arrival in Peshawar, which he predicted might shortly be looked for. At that time such news circulating through an excitable population like that of Delhi might have done much harm; but it is believed that most of his notes fell into the hands of police.[71]

Mr H. was an interesting case as he was already a troubled political subject because he was an Irishman. He became a menace because he was bitterly rancorous about the British government and had called upon Muslims to aid Russians. Moreover, Mr H.'s conversion to Islam gained him many supporters. The authorities were alarmed and used insanity as a device to suppress any kind of resistance. There are other cases as well that tell us that the colonial government often declared people mad in order to suppress any kind of possible confrontation. The violence of colonialism is illustrated in the following cases:

> A man as sent in who was found sitting on a bridge abusing every passerby. His weak point is, that he wrote to the Queen, he says, because the Government was not capable of ruling Kabul and by the Kyber, but if the charge was given over to him, he would settle matters to her satisfaction. On every subject he is quite rational.[72]

Another patient imagines himself to be Alagmir come to life again.[73]

[...] Imrit says that he is descended from Sen dynasty, that he has given India on contract of 80 years to the English, after which time he will drive them out and divide the country between the Russian and Chinese.[74]

---

[71] The Annual Report of the Lunatic Asylums of the Punjab for the Year 1877, NAI.

[72] The Annual Report of the Lunatic Asylums of the Punjab for the Year 1881, NAI.

[73] The Annual Report of the Lunatic Asylums of the Punjab for the Year 1881, NAI.

[74] The Annual Report of the Lunatic Asylums the Punjab for the Year 1883, NAI.

Habib Shah, a dirzy. His delusion is that he is the last of the Mughal dynasty, and has been sent by Nizam-ud-din Auliya to take possession of the throne of Delhi.[75]

Frantz Fanon argued that 'these disorders take various forms. Sometimes they are visible as states of agitation which sometimes turn into rages; sometimes deep depression and tonic immobility with many attempted suicides; or sometimes finally anxiety states with tears, lamentations, and appeals for mercy'.[76] Colonialism generated deep-seated fears and the most imminent of them was losing one's independence. These were lamentations and appeals of mercy which were mixed with illusions of independence. The colonial state ingeniously invented a mechanism to curtail freedom of the so-called delinquent subjects. Mental hospitals can definitely be regarded as one of the state-invented devices that aimed to keep troubled populations in control.

Psychiatric power became much fuzzier in the colonial milieu. Nationalist feelings continued to find place in the Agra Mental Hospital records:

Baijnath—32—Ahir—Admitted to the Agra Mental Hospital on 29.4.38—Schizophrenia—Aggressive—claims to be khilafat worker and law breaker—refuses food—uncontrollable—Confused cleaning— Incoherent cleaning—Dull cleaning—sensible cleaning—He struck patient Mattri—excitable no work—irritable no work—quiet— Discharged on 26-3-42.[77]

Baijnath remained in the Agra Mental Hospital for four years. His certificate indicates that he was 'aggressive and claimed to be a khila-fat worker and law breaker'. He was diagnosed with schizophrenia and the two words which describe his behaviour are 'aggressive' and

[75] The Annual Report of the Lunatic Asylums the Punjab for the Year 1883, NAI.

[76] Frantz Fanon, *The Wretched of the Earth*, translated by Constance Farrington (New York: Grove Press, 1963), 280.

[77] A short summary of the case is discussed here. The complete case history is available in Appendix no. 4, Case no. 19; Register no. 61, the Agra Mental Hospital, NAI.

'uncontrollable'. No symptom related to the disease itself has been noted. It is difficult to ascertain the extent to which Baijnath suffered from insanity. During his stay at the hospital, the terms 'confused', 'incoherent', 'dull', and in 'sensible' were used interchangeably to describe his condition. Except for one incidence of violence, Baijnath's behaviour was within the boundaries of 'control'.

The authorities saw such individuals as problematic and sent them to mental hospitals. The case notes indicate that these 'madmen' (if they were at all mad) had 'illusions of independence'[78] and thus became a matter of concern for the authorities. In the very ravings and gibberish of these so-called madmen, one sees a desire for independence and the level of alienation they experienced. The following case note shows that not only nationalism but also communalism permeates the records of the period:

> Khan Bahadur & Abdul Rahaman—55—Admitted to the Agra Mental Hospital on 29-4-38 Contractor Roorki—Paranoia N.A.D—suffering from delusions that Congress wants to kill him that he has had instructions from God that he wants to kill all Hindus who were congressmen, that an attempt was made on his life when travelling to Sahranpur. Dr Rizvi Medical Officer Civil Hospitals Roorke. The wheel of the car came off. This incident is known to be true but the patients says that the Dr Rizvi tried to kill him—while under observation he would only have one particular mohmmaden cook to prepare his meals as he stated that others would poison him. He feared persecution from the chairman of municipality R S Muthura Dass and therefore ward off doors of his quarters. He states that he has no fear as life is drawing to close—god has given him sufficient strength to kill all the Hindus—refuses to talk says that he free from mental trouble—no work—Reads Books—Discharged under 31 on 26-3-42.[79]

Khan Bahadur suffered from delusions that were part of mass paranoia. Communalist feelings were common and affected individuals in

---

[78] Kala, Sarin, and Jain, 'The Psychiatrist's Partition': 3.

[79] A short summary of the case is discussed here. The complete case history is available in Appendix no. 5, Case no 52; Register no. 61, the Agra Mental Hospital, NAI.

different manners. It can be argued that it was the 'madness of communalism' that made Khan Bahadur hallucinate. His acts of openly confessing to killing all Hindus belonging to the Congress party would have alerted the community members. Bahadur stayed in the hospital for four years and was declared sane under Section 31 by the Visitors in Charge of the hospital.

Vaughan has aptly asserted,

> The language of the psyche was and is a powerful one, whether it is wielded by professional psychiatrists, or by local communities defining who is, and who is not, behaving according to accepted norms. It is also a language which can be used for a range of political purposes. Colonial psychiatrists often (but not always) used it to define the normal native as abnormal—a rather alarming notion, but one which had some political utility when colonial nationalism appeared to be running out of control.[80]

The madness of the state and the madness of the subject differed because of the underlying difference of structure of power and coercion. The colonial state's irrationalism was streamlined and rationalized through the creation of the psychiatric power that was backed up by the whole legal, medical, and judicial systems. The state did not shy away from the use of these structures (if required) to treat madness and delinquencies.

The Rich and the Middle Classes

In the nineteenth century, lunatic asylums in colonial India were filled by the mad and the 'debauched' (ganja, charas, and opium smokers along with the 'others' who are seen as deviant, such as faqirs). Historians agree that most of the inmates in asylums were picked up from the streets by the police. Nile Green even contends that nineteenth-century lunatic asylums should be placed within the ambit of larger colonial anti-vagrant policies. This began to change by the twentieth century when the middle class started utilizing the asylums. The records (especially the case registers) show that the middle classes had emerged as an important force. This change was the result of several complex processes.

---

[80] Megan Vaughan, 'Introduction', in *Psychiatry and Empire*, edited by Sloan Mahone and Megan Vaughan (New York: Palgrave Macmillan, 2007), 15.

B. B. Misra argues that with the establishment of British rule in India, fundamental changes took place in the field of political and economic administration. These changes along with progress in education and technology created fertile conditions for the emergence of the middle class in India.[81] The term 'middle class' remains elusive since no succinct definition of the term exists. Misra did not define the term in his work and stated that 'most of us, without any aid of a specialist, understand what we mean, when we use it in our everyday conversation.'[82] Sanjay Joshi in his work on the middle class critiques Misra's arguments and has posited that 'important social, economic and political changes accompanying British rule in India undoubtedly presented new opportunities to educated men and a little later women as well. But ultimately being middle class, in India, as elsewhere, was a project of self-fashioning.'[83] Joshi emphasizes on the cultural projection of the middle class that implicitly tried to create a separate identity by differentiating it from the upper class and the lower class.[84] This project of self-fashioning had in its bag the projection of the so-called scientific outlook. Deepak Kumar argues that 'the Indians, especially the neo-elites, were worried about what the British thought of them. So efforts were made right from the days of Raja Rammohun Roy to project certain Indian traditions and ideas as fully compatible with and not opposed to modern science.'[85] These justifications of compatibility—by the neo-elites and the middle class—gradually declined since the middle class with its claims for rationality and 'science' gradually accepted the developments in the fields of science and medicine.

At least in the case of psychiatry, it may be argued that the acceptance was the result of complex processes at work. The asylums in nineteenth-century India were more or less 'reformed jails' that were made especially

---

[81] B. B. Misra, *The Indian Middle Classes: Their Growth in Modern Times* (London: Oxford University Press, 1961), 10–12.

[82] Misra, *The Indian Middle Classes*, 10–12.

[83] Sanjay Joshi, *Fractured Modernity: Making of a Middle Class in Colonial North India* (New Delhi: Oxford University Press, 2001), 6.

[84] Joshi, *Fractured Modernity*, 7–8.

[85] Deepak Kumar, *Science and the Raj: A Study of British India* (New Delhi: Oxford University Press, 2006), 271.

for the insane, with an emphasis on the moral management system. It is not to deny that they provided relief to the homeless and some of the people actually suffering from insanity, but the lunatic asylum's intended goal was to house the 'dangerous' classes. These characteristics of nineteenth-century asylums should be understood by placing them within the larger context of colonialism. These prison-like features would have been a significant reason why the emerging middle class were apathetic towards these places. Nonetheless, by the twentieth century, attempts were made to medicalize and professionalize the psychiatric infrastructure. As discussed in Chapter 2, these attempts were not very successful, but they signalled change and altered the psychiatric infrastructure. The colonial state attempted to cater to the emerging middle classes by providing them with special provisions. Separate rooms were designed to treat the Indian 'gentlemen' and 'ladies' who could pay for their stay. These rooms were situated separately so that the 'noisy' and 'troublesome' sections of the insane population incarcerated in the asylums could be kept away.

The Agra Mental Hospital's case registers mirror an increasing use of the asylum spaces by different classes. The traditional elites such as zamindars resided in these hospitals and the middle classes also availed of the newly reformed psychiatric services available in these hospitals. In the following subsection, certain illustrative cases belonging to categories such as the rich, the middle class, and the petty bourgeoisie will be discussed.

***

Raghu Nath Rai—50—Hindu—Zamindar—Ghazipur—Admitted to the Agra Mental Hospital on 21-8-38—dementia—Old Age—violent and abusive—dirty in habits—remains naked—tears clothes—damages walls and cell badly—sleeps and eats sparingly—dull—no work—Bromide mix—died of maniacal excitement on 29-1-39.[86]

Raghu Nath Rai was a 50-year-old zamindar. He was diagnosed with age-related dementia and stayed in the Agra Mental Hospital for a

[86] A short summary of the case is discussed here. The complete case history is available in Appendix no. 6, Case no 54; Register no. 61, the Agra Mental Hospital, NAI.

span of about five months. His refusal to participate in any sort of work would have contributed to his characterization of 'bad behaviour'. Work, as discussed before (Chapter 3), was considered pertinent in assessing insanity and its recovery. Raghu Nath Rai was given sedatives such as bromide mix, but it did not help much as he died of 'maniacal excitement'. Rai was described as 'violent', 'abusive', 'dirty', and 'maniacal'. Words like 'abusive', 'filthy', and 'violent' have a much longer history of being used in the colonial discourse to describe the insanity of 'natives'. What is worth noticing here is the fact that these became an integral part of psychiatric repertoire by the twentieth century. They were internalized by Indians who became the Superintendents in Charge of the mental hospitals and other similar medical authorities who identified and certified insanity in the twentieth century. James H. Mills in his work shows that the use of such terms justified the treatment regimes in colonial India. He states that 'whether the patient was violent and demonstrative or feeble and distracted, the medical officer would attempt to control and manipulate his/her behaviour through a series of assaults on his/her mind and body'.[87]

Rai was regarded as an old and demented patient. On the eve of Independence, life expectancy at birth was 32.5 years.[88] Anyone who lived after the expected 32.5 years was considered to be old. However, as we know today, there are only minute chances of people suffering from age-related dementia at the age of 50. These odd probabilities are only possible with the early onset of the Alzheimer's disease. There is a serious dearth of scholarship on the history of ageing in the colonial period. Lawrence Cohen has worked on the notions of senility and family in postcolonial India.[89] However, in his work he has tried to look at the ideas related to age and senility in the colonial discourse. Cohen describes that the colonial concerns were mainly related to

[87] James H. Mills, 'Reforming the Indian: Treatment Regimes in the Lunatic Asylums of British India, 1857–1880', *Indian Economic and Social History Review*, vol. 36, no. 4 (1999): 422.

[88] B. R. Tomlinson, *The Economy of Modern India 1860–1947* (New York: Cambridge, 1993), 7.

[89] Lawrence Cohen, *No Aging in India: Modernity, Senility and the Family* (New Delhi: Oxford University Press, 1998).

British families in India. He cited a 1907 health manual for British families in India which stated, 'There is little doubt that the exposure of Europeans to the effects of continued tropical heat during a series of years produces a debilitated condition of the system, consequent of blood degeneration, favorable to brain softening.'[90] Cohen further noted, 'Throughout the nineteenth century, attention to corporeal decay and its management intensifies as a European mode of understanding Indian difference and the biopolitics of empire increasingly encompass Reason, no longer invulnerable to precocious decline. Indian minds are naturally soft and, though not in danger of sudden softening, are in a sense congenially senile.'[91]

This construction of age as equivalent to senility is not the only problem of the colonial records. Mills has, in fact, shown through his work on the nineteenth-century case notes of the Lucknow Lunatic Asylum that 'of the 721 notes, 508 have ages which are entered as multiples of five. In other words about 70 percent of the patients were entered as being 15, 20, 25, 30 and so on years old upon admission. This suggests that a process of estimation was at work on the part of the medical officer in the case note'.[92] In the absence of birth records, calculation of age itself became a difficult task. Much was left upon the medical officers and on the family members of the patients. More and more patients during the twentieth century were brought to the hospital by their relatives. The colonial legal framework along with medical discourses on ageing and dementia created an infrastructure for the children of rich old parents (for example, zamindars such as Raghu Nath Rai) to declare the latter insane and incarcerate them within the hospital walls.

Carol Berkenkotter asserts that 'from a discursive perspective the clinical case history is actually a double narrative. The patient's story of his or her narrative of personal experiences, is subsumed into the narrative pattern and thought style of clinical psychiatry'.[93] The stories of

[90] William Moore, *A Manual of Family Medicine and Hygiene in India*, 7th ed. (Delhi: Sri Satguru, 1989 [1907]), cited in Cohen, *No Aging in India*, 22.

[91] Cohen, *No Aging in India*, 22.

[92] James H. Mills, *Madness, Cannabis and Colonialism: The 'Native-Only' Lunatic Asylums of British India, 1857–1900* (Basingstoke: Macmillan, 2000), 16.

[93] Berkenkotter, *Patient Tales*, 2.

the patients' families often took precedence over patients' experiences. Once declared 'mad', patients lost the credibility of being rational beings. In this scenario, the narratives of family members along with modern discourses on insanity created a volatile possibility of the patients (especially those considered problematic, unproductive, and old) being sent (temporarily or permanently) to mental hospitals.

S. N. Ray—50 years—Brahmin—Lecturer in Physics—admitted to the Agra Mental Hospital on 12.1.37—Paranoid Dementia—suffered from dysentery—excited and destructive—no work—recovers and weight gain—tears clothes—fights with fellow inmates and attendant—put on sulfosin—violent and naked—tears bedding and clothes—no work—ECT (21 shocks biweek)—irrelevant talk—mitral regulation—murmurs—gradually weakening—expired on 15.12.51.[94]

S. N. Ray was a 50-year-old lecturer in physics. He spent about 11 years of his life in the Agra Mental Hospital, but his case notes are only available from 1946 to 1951.[95] He was diagnosed with paranoid dementia, which means that age-related dementia was fused with paranoia. Wright has described paranoia as 'systematised delusional insanity'.[96] Eventually, in the twentieth century, paranoia became a sub-category of schizophrenia known as paranoid schizophrenia. Schizophrenia as a category became reified in Western psychiatry. However, dementia and paranoia's clubbing together here shows a palpable link between ageing and senility. Ray has been described as 'destructive', 'violent', and 'unproductive'. He smacked the attendant Ram Narain and quarrelled with a fellow inmate, Jasbeer Singh. Singh in turn hit Ray. Ray was not only 'quarrelsome' but was still portrayed as 'destructive'. His behaviour left little possibility of him ever gaining his freedom.

[94] A short summary of the case is discussed here. The complete case history is available in Appendix no. 7, Case no. 8; Register nos 58–59, the Agra Mental Hospital, NAI.

[95] Registers 58–59 are in continuation with the old registers. The old registers are not available. Therefore, Mr Ray's case notes are only available from the year 1946.

[96] Overbeck-Wright, *Lunacy in India*, 106.

By the twentieth century, the entire mechanism of treatment related to insanity had taken a different turn. As discussed in Chapter 3, shock therapy and fever therapy were widely used. Sulfosin therapy was one of the fever therapies. It was believed that a high-grade fever would cure insanity. We find from the notes that sulfosin therapy was largely unsuccessful since Ray showed no signs of improvement. It was stated that he 'tears all the beddings (blanket and Dari)'. Words such as 'excited', 'violent', 'abusive', and 'naked' have been used. Ray was given ECT on a regular basis from 25 August to 27 October 1948. He was given 21 shocks biweekly. This treatment resumed on 19 November and lasted till 13 December 1948. ECT was used for the first time to give shocks by Italian neuropsychiatrist Ugo Cerletti in 1937, and the ECT machine was first introduced in India in the Agra Mental Hospital in 1945.[97] The newly transferred technology was used to cure Ray's insanity. The case records state that Ray was 'manageable when he is getting electricity otherwise he is very destructive and mischievous.'[98] Thus, we can see that ECT made patients manageable. The therapy continued while Ray's health saw a marked decline. He was weak, anemic, and feverish. The rigorous punitive treatment of ECT would have been an added factor to Ray's failing mental and physical health. Ray died on 15 December 1951. His death was ascribed to heart disease. Visits by relatives are usually mentioned on the side of the pages on which the recorded histories of the patients are available. In the case of S. N. Ray, there was no mention of relatives visiting. Ray met a lonesome death at the age of 61.

Ismail Khan—35—Muslim—railway service—admitted to the Agra Mental Hospital on 30-3-38—Melancholia—delusions of having committed unpardonable sins of having insulted great men—dull and depressed—suicidal—depressed—cleaning—depressed—factory— sensible—factory—depressed—brick making—better than before— improving—discharged on 18-6-40.[99]

[97] The Annual Report on the Mental Hospital in the United Provinces for the Year 1945, NAI.

[98] Case no. 8; Register nos 58–9, the Agra Mental Hospital, NAI.

[99] A short summary of the case is discussed here. The complete case history is available in Appendix no. 8, Case no 7; Register no. 61, the Agra Mental Hospital, NAI.

Ismail Khan was a 35-year-old railway employee. He was in the Agra Mental Hospital for a period of two years and three months. Khan was described as 'delusional', 'depressed', and 'suicidal'. He had 'delusions of insulting great men and of committing unpardonable sins'.[100] His delusions were understood as the source of his depression. Khan was in government service and an enquiry, therefore, was made into his condition from his fellow worker, Nannhy Khan (driver block). His fellow workers and friends visited him during the period of his stay. Khan's participation and involvement in the factory (where useable items were manufactured) and in brick making were interpreted as signs of recovery. Mills rightly points out that 'work was central to the modes of treating the Indian inmate as it became the means and measure of "recovery" in the patient'.[101] He was relieved under section 33 of the Indian Lunacy Act, according to which 'when any relative or friend of a lunatic detained in any asylum … is desirous that such lunatic shall be delivered over to his care and custody',[102] and thus the patient was released. Khan was more fortunate than the other two cases that have been discussed previously since his participation and family support paved the way to his freedom.

'Melancholia', which Ismail Khan was diagnosed with, is a term that has its origins in Graeco-Roman medicine. According to contemporary understanding, the term signifies depression. Melancholia according to Graeco-Roman medicine was a disorder rising due to humoral imbalances. This term continued to be a part of psychiatric vocabulary up till the nineteenth century. Roy Porter highlights while discussing case histories from the Hippocratic writings that 'delusional melancholia have said to arise from black bile collecting in the liver and rising to the head, [and] involved a condition which "usually attacks abroad, if a person is travelling a lonely road somewhere, and fear seizes him"'.[103]

---

[100] A short summary of the case is discussed here. The complete case history is available in Appendix no. 8, Case no 7; Register no. 61, the Agra Mental Hospital, NAI.

[101] Mills, *Madness, Cannabis and Colonialism*, 120.

[102] The Indian Lunacy Act No. IV of 1912, NAI.

[103] Roy Porter, *Madness: A Brief History* (Oxford: Oxford University Press, 2002), 43.

Berrios has remarked that by the nineteenth century 'some old categories (e.g. delirium) emerged unchanged; others, such as melancholia and mania were totally refurbished with new clinical meaning'.[104] Melancholia was thus reconstituted as depression during the period. The term was 'applied to the lowness of spirits of persons suffering under disease'.[105] Berrios pointed out that 'British psychiatry took longer to catch up, and continued treating the same groups of disorders as 'melancholia'; witness to this is the famous 'Nomenclature of Diseases' drawn up by a joint committee appointed by the Royal College of Physicians of London in 1906.[106] Emil Kraepelin was the German psychiatrist who used the term 'manic-depressive disorder' to describe cases of those who underwent depression and phases of exaltation. W. S. J. Shaw mentioned in his work that 'Kraepelin suggested the name of "manic-depressive" insanity, cases belonging to this group were designated "mania", "melancholia" according as the symptom of excitement or exaltation suggested mania, or depression melancholia [sic]'.[107] This manic-depressive disorder was later in the twentieth century reconstituted as depression and as bipolar disorder. The use of the term 'melancholia' reflects not only the way in which Ismail Khan's case history was constructed but also exposes the backwardness of colonial psychiatry. The use of antiquated terms points towards delayed development of modern psychiatry in India.

> Gopal Narian—18—Kayath—Student—Admitted to the Agra Mental Hospital on 30.9.38—confusional insanity—Business worry—explosive and excitable—wants to marry Kamla Jharia famous radio singer—has grandious ideas about himself—sensible—quite sensible—discharged on 30.6.39.[108]

---

[104] Berrios, *History of Mental Symptoms*, 17.

[105] Berrios, *History of Mental Symptoms*, 299.

[106] Berrios, *History of Mental Symptoms*, 300.

[107] W. S. Jagoe Shaw, *A Clinical Handbook of Mental Diseases; for the Use of Students and Medical Practitioners in India* (Calcutta; Butterworth & Co. Limited, 1925), 27.

[108] A short summary of the case is discussed here. The complete case history is available in Appendix no. 9, Case no. 63; Register no. 61, the Agra Mental Hospital, NAI.

Gopal Narian was an 18-year-old student. He stayed in the Agra Mental Hospital for the period of nine months. Narian was depicted as 'explosive' and 'excitable' in the medical certificate and was diagnosed with confusional insanity. The cause of his insanity was business worry. There is no mention of business in the case notes of Narian, however. This reflects the pressure of filling up the columns without much serious consideration. Nonetheless, he was described as 'sensible' after a few days of his stay. The word sensible was 'replaced' by the word 'quite sensible' by March of 1939. Narian was released on 30 June of the same year. Berrios argues that 'since the 1860s confusion has referred to the defect in the organisation of ideas found in delirium, severe depression and other insanities'.[109] W. S. J. Shaw described confusional insanity as follows:

> The group of mental diseases ... characterised by sudden onset and a tendency to early recovery. The striking symptoms are *confusion* and *delirium*. The term confusion means a state of disorientation in the sphere of time, space and personality ... The term delirium may be defined as a clouded state of consciousness due to a definite cause of which ceases with the operation of the cause.[110]

The 'confusion' was in Narian's delusion of marrying a famous radio singer. The toxic state of delirium refers to his state of being in love.

Narian belonged to a family of advocates whose faith in modern science and medicine is reflected in the fact that they sent their 'wayward' teenage son to a mental hospital. Historians of psychiatry in England, North America, and other Western European countries have delineated the role of families in not only decision-making but also in participating (if not intervening) on an equal front with the psychiatrist. The care and cure offered to their 'insane' relatives was thus a result of a joint venture.[111] Akihito Suzuki has looked at family and insanity in England.

---

[109] Berrios, *History of Mental Symptoms*, 233.

[110] Shaw, *A Clinical Handbook of Mental Diseases*, 52.

[111] Wright, *Mental Disability in Victorian England*; Patricia E. Prestwich, 'Family Strategies and Medical Power: "Voluntary" Committals in a Parisian Asylum, 1876–1914', *Journal of Social History*, vol. 27, no. 4 (1994): 799–818; Akihito Suzuki, *Madness at Home: The Psychiatrist, the Patient and the Family in England, 1820–1860* (California: University of California Press, 2006).

He has pointed out that 'practising psychiatrists were often integrated into family affairs, largely playing an ancillary, if not always subordinate, part.'[112] Feminist historians have also pointed out that women were often sent to asylums by their husbands in order to exert control over their behaviour and lives.[113]

In the Indian context, the limitations of the available archival material have impeded historians from looking into these connections further. New sources would have to be recovered in order to comprehend doctor–patient–family relationships and networks. Narian's case provides us with an imperative entry point since his case notes reveal nothing related to his so-called 'mental illness'. His teenage feelings for the famous radio singer Kamla Jharia led to his incarceration in the hospital. Radio was introduced in India in August 1927 but it was not until 1935 that radio broadcasting became a regular thing.[114] Partha Sarthi Gupta avers that the actual number of transmission 'licences at the end of 1932 was 8557, which had risen to 92,782 at the end of 1939'.[115] The growing popularity of radio enchanted this teenage boy. Narian, after his sojourn of nine months at the mental hospital, was discharged under section 32 of the 1912 Indian Lunacy Act. This section stated:

> A lunatic detained in any asylum under a reception order, made on petition, shall be discharged if the person on whose petition the reception order was made so applies in writing to the person in charge of the asylum: provided that no lunatic shall be discharged under the provisions of sub-section ... if the officer-in-charge of the asylum certifies in writing that the lunatic is dangerous and unfit to be at large.[116]

Accordingly, Narian's family must have requested for his release. The middle-class families used the asylum spaces for control and correction.

---

[112] Suzuki, *Madness at Home*, 91.

[113] For feminist perspectives, see Showalter, *The Female Malady*; Ripa, *Women and Madness*.

[114] Partha Sarathi Gupta, *Power, Politics and the People: Studies in British Imperialism and Indian Nationalism* (New Delhi: Permanent Black, 2001), 448.

[115] Gupta, *Power, Politics and the People*, 449.

[116] The Indian Lunacy Act No. IV of 1912, NAI.

Their ability to pay helped them in exerting control on those who were considered to be difficult or to abandon those who were considered unproductive. This is not to deny that patients with severe mental illnesses were also sent to the hospitals because they could not be handled properly at home or they became a source of shame.

Misra has argued that the middle class included a wide array of professions from professors to merchants and from clerks to shopkeepers.[117] The term 'middle class' elides the fact that shopkeepers and lower-rung of government servants lived on the edge. Patch, the Superintendent of the Lahore Mental Hospital, remarked:

> It was found that the government was incurring considerable loss by accessing the maintenance rates of patient at Rs. 16 per month, so it was raised to Rs. 20 with effect to 1st January 1924 ... So long as the state pays, relations are quite indifferent as to how long a patient is left in an asylum or what becomes of him ... it became a matter for the application of the most elementary form of economics, because it is very much cheaper to keep a half witted father or brother locked in a dark room or tied to a tree than to pay Rs. 20 per month towards the maintenance at the local asylum. As a natural consequence, therefore, numerous requests were received for urgent representations were made for the discharge of patients who have been in the institution for years.[118]

While some families could afford to pay the increased amount, others failed to pay. Ernst has pointed out that 'the income related scale of fees implemented at the Yeravda Asylum in Bombay in the early twentieth century indicates differentiation between European, Parsi and other Indian patients.'[119] There were many sub-classes amongst the middle classes. The rich were also not a single class since there were neo-elites and traditional elites. Some of these traditional elites were able to maintain their status and wealth while the influence of others declined. Nonetheless, this section of the chapter has shown that there

---

[117] Misra, *The Indian Middle Classes*, 12–13.

[118] Patch, *A Critical Review of the Punjab Mental Hospitals*, 78–9.

[119] Waltraud Ernst, 'Madness and Colonial Spaces British India, 1800–1947', in *Madness, Architecture and the Built Environment*, edited by Leslie Topp, James Moran, and Jonathan Andrews (London: Routledge, 2007), 220.

was a marked increase in the general population who utilized psychiatric services in the twentieth century.

***

Asylum records show that fewer women were incarcerated in the Indian asylums compared to men. On the one hand, statistical data allowed questioning of the larger assumption that in India insanity was a female malady. On the other hand, it has been argued that diagnosis and categorization of insanity in women were viewed through a gender-biased lens. Throughout the nineteenth century, the asylums were abodes of the poor and the vagrant. These institutions were utilized to 'shut off' the homeless who were regarded by the state as a public nuisance. Nonetheless, the lunatic asylums offered shelter and food to the poor and the 'idiots'. There was a transformation of this trend by the twentieth century, when the middle classes and the rich began using these institutions. The state made an effort to privatize and popularize these places. The case notes of patients belonging to the newly emergent middle class reflect how the stories of patients and their relatives gained epistemological meanings. Places such as the lunatic asylums provided spaces to the state and the families to 'shut off' people who were 'difficult'. Families sequestered their wayward sons, 'senile' fathers, and rebellious wives. The colonial state not only incarcerated the vagrants and the poor but sometimes also locked away delinquent subjects. This included people who imagined themselves to be emperors or empresses or individuals who had actually participated in the freedom struggle.

This chapter tried to bring to the fore certain important illustrative cases. As these cases are illustrative, they cannot be generalized. The categories discussed here overlap each other and thus cannot be divided into watertight compartments. Attempts have been made to show through the study of the case notes and the case histories how the state, individuals, and society at large made use of the psychiatric structure. It has attempted to reveal the latent motives of the three main actors—the state, the individuals, and the families. It has, in its own way, destabilized the above-mentioned psychiatric umbrella categories in order to unravel the therapeutic as well as the coercive side of psychiatric science.

It is also imperative to state that under colonialism the distinction between the civil and the criminally insane was often blurred. This was due to several reasons. The civil liberties of the subject remained at the mercy of the colonial state. Mental institutions throughout the period were extremely unpopular and 'respectable' men or women never willingly admitted their relatives into these pagal khanas. The stigma attached with incarceration in these institutions was widespread since civil patients were often treated like criminal lunatics.

5 Indigenous Traditions, Modernity, and Madness

In some parts of Bengal frog soup is a favourite remedy for insanity, and among the Feringee—the degenerate descendants of the Portuguese—a live frog fastened on the top of the shaven scalp is reputed to be a sovereign remedy for extracting the morbid heat which causes mania.[1]

There already exist some major scholarly contributions in the field of the history of psychiatry and mental hospitals in colonial India. However, the impact of Western psychiatry on traditional healing practices has been overlooked. Western medical ideas were sometimes amalgamated, segregated, filtered, and appropriated by the vaidyas and *hakims* (practitioners of indigenous forms of medicine) according to the needs of the time. Certain key psychiatric concepts

[1] Sir James Clark's Enquiry as to the Care and the Treatment of Lunatics, Home Dept./Public Branch, File Nos 22–3, 19 December 1868, NAI.

had long and interesting afterlives while others could not survive. These hybrid practices reflect not only the wide circulation of knowledge but also the impulses of the medical markets[2] that recast traditional medicine in a modern garb.

This chapter is a preliminary investigation into the indigenous ways of dealing with and healing madness. The spread and dissemination of Western medical knowledge led to the reshaping of some of the Ayurvedic concepts of mental illness. Historians working on modern Ayurveda have delineated the differences between ancient and modern Ayurveda. Nationalist acquisitions of the Western medical discourses on psychiatric diseases often reflect gender biases and communal hostilities. Extending this scholarship further, it is argued here that looking at the colonial and nationalist milieus is imperative to comprehend and contextualize the resurgence of Ayurvedic medical traditions in

[2] The concept of medical market here refers to competition between the Western and the Eastern practices of medicine in colonial India. Canonical systems such as Ayurveda and Unani were forced to modernize themselves due to widespread attacks made by the colonial state on such practices. The advent of colonialism also led to commercialization of medical practices and goods. Plural Indian medical practices when faced with competition from Western medicine were forced to reinvent and recast themselves. The colonial state relegated Indian systems of healing as quackery and superstition. This led to the reshaping and filtrations of Western ideas. For details, see Kavita Sivaramakrishnan, *Old Potions, New Bottles: Recasting Indigenous Medicine in Colonial Punjab, 1850–1945* (Hyderabad: Orient Longman, 2006); Projit Bihari Mukharji, *Nationalizing the Body: The Medical Market, Print and Daktari Medicine* (London: Anthem Press, 2009); Madhuri Sharma, *Indigenous and Western Medicine in Colonial India* (New Delhi: Foundation Books, 2012); Guy Attwell, *Refiguring Unani Tibb: Plural Healing in Late Colonial India* (Hyderabad: Orient Longman, 2007); and Seema Alavi, *Islam and Healing: Loss and Recovery of an Indo-Muslim Medical Tradition, 1600–1900* (Palgrave Macmillan, 2008). More generally, the medical market is understood from the early 1980s as a phenomenon marked by commercialization and consumerism of medicine. The concept has undergone various turns. For details, see Roy Porter, *Health for Sale: Quackery in England 1660–1850* (Manchester: Manchester University Press, 1989), Harold J. Cook, 'Good Advice and Little Medicine: The Professional Authority of Early Modern English Physicians', *Journal of British Studies* 33, no. 1 (1994): 1–31.

late nineteenth- and early twentieth-century north India. Based on an examination of Hindi medical advice literature, which primarily includes books, pamphlets, and periodicals, this chapter locates the history of madness outside the asylum walls.

Recasting Traditions

The ancient Ayurvedic texts provide a detailed discussion regarding the diagnosis and prognosis of unmada or severe psychiatric illness. Mitchell Weiss points out that according to the *Caraka Samhita*, there exist endogenous (*nija-*) unmada and exogenous (*agantu-*) unmada.[3] The former refers to a class of disorders resulting from an imbalance of one or combination of the three pathogenic bodily elements or dosas. The agantu categories refer to a non-physiologic mechanism that is external to human. He further points out that according to 'Susruta, Vagbhata, and other traditional medical authors unmada could occur due to suffering and a hardship (*dukha*) and also be effect of powerful drugs (*visa*).'[4] The Buddhist concept that dukha or suffering is part of human existence differs from the Ayurvedic concept which regards dukha as aberration to human existence.

The agantu categories refer to spiritual, magical, and other religious factors leading to mental illnesses. The diseases that could not be attributed to any dosa were explained through the supernatural belief system. Weiss discusses in detail that 'the onset of an episode of agantu-unmada is typically marked by a specific or cognitive abnormality, including various types of hallucinations, delusions, and/derealisation phenomena associated with a particular bhuta. Parts of the lunar fortnight (*tithi*) are also associated with specific bhutas, although these may vary from one text to another.'[5] Horacio Fabrega points out that it can also be conceptualized as 'metaphysical' since alongside practical considerations it also drew on 'unseen but real' and '"other than natural"

---

[3] Mitchell G. Weiss, 'Critical Study of Unmada in Early Sanskrit Literature: An Analysis of Ayurvedic Psychiatry with Reference to Present-day Diagnostic Concepts', unpublished doctoral thesis, University of Pennsylvania, 1977, 1

[4] Weiss, 'Critical Study of Unmada', 1.

[5] Weiss, 'Critical Study of Unmada', 112–13.

agencies (spirits, demons, ancestors, witchcraft)' to explain supposedly 'enigmatic' conditions associated with emotional and behavioural
problems.[6]

A number of hospitals were established for mentally ill patients
during the reign of Ashoka.[7] During the medieval period, Najabuddin
Unhammad (1222), an Indian physician, explained seven types of
mental illnesses: 'Sauda-a-Tabee (Schizophrenia); Muree Sauda
(depression); Ishk (delusion of love); Nisyan (Organic mental disorder); Haziyan (paranoid state); Malikholia-a-maraki (delirium)'.[8]
There was a mental hospital at Dhar in Madhya Pradesh which was
established during the period of Mahmood Khalji (1436–1469).[9]
There is no proper study on insanity and its treatment in medieval
India. Micheal W. Dols's work interestingly throws light on how insanity and its treatment were conceptualized in Islamic societies. Dols
points out that 'the special provision for the insane is a remarkable
aspect of the Islamic hospital. 'Unlike the earlier Byzantine hospitals,
the Islamic hospitals invariably included wards for men and women
who were mentally ill ... A maristan [here refers to 'bimaristan' or
hospital] was certainly founded by Ibn Tulun in Egypt in AD 872–3,
and it appears to have provided for the insane.'[10] He also explains that
during the period it was believed,

Insanity was a disturbance or dysfunction of the brain, which controlled
mental activity and emotions. The functioning of the brain, and the body
in general, depended upon the proper mixture of the humours and their
qualities, so that the treatment of any illness was aimed at the restoration of the balance of these humours. It may be said that this somatic
approach created the concept of 'mental illness'.[11]

---

[6] Horacio Fabrega Jr., *History of Mental Illness in India: A Cultural Psychiatry Retrospective* (Delhi: Motilal Banarasidas, 2009), 320.

[7] S. Haque Nizamie and Nishant Goyal, 'History of Psychiatry in India', *Indian Journal of Psychiatry*, vol. 52, no. 7, (2010): 7.

[8] Nizamie and Goyal, 'History of Psychiatry in India': 7.

[9] Nizamie and Goyal, 'History of Psychiatry in India': 7.

[10] Micheal W. Dols, 'Insanity and Its Treatment in Islamic Society', *Medical History*, vol. 31 (1987): 3.

[11] Dols, 'Insanity and Its Treatment in Islamic Society': 4.

Western medicine appropriated many Islamic ideas of insanity and its treatment. Dols points out,

> Judging by the medieval medical texts, the doctors apparently paid close attention to the patient's regimen; the 'non-naturals', especially exercise, a restful environment, and ample sleep, should be studied and adjusted, so that the patient's daily life would be conducive to recovery. Treatment included baths, fomentations (particularly to the head), compresses, bandaging, and massage with various oils. Bloodletting, leeches, cupping, and cautery also appear to have been used ... The drugs included purgatives, emetics, digestives, and sedatives, especially opium.[12]

These ideas when reconceptualized became the basis of the moral management in nineteenth century.

The Islamic concept of insanity also had a considerable impact on the Ayurvedic notion of madness and its treatment. Weiss argues that the idea of a continuous linear tradition of Ayurveda needs to be questioned as diagnostic pulse feeling and the therapeutic use of mixtures with calcinated mercury may be traced back to Persian and Arabic influences which were later introduced into Ayurvedic practice.[13] Neither the Indian nor the Western medical systems acknowledged the debt they owe to Islamic ideas about the mind, body, and healing which truly transformed our understanding of insanity.

India has inherited an eclectic tradition of healing that primarily includes Ayurvedic, Unani, Buddhist, Siddha, and tribal medicine, which has significantly contributed to the curative notions of well-being. Insanity was and continues to be treated in innumerable dargarhs, temples, and shrines. Waltraud Ernst argues that medical practices based on the eminent classical traditions of Ayurveda and Unani continue to be relevant in India. Colonial modernity disparaged of these notions of healing and curing madness. Medical practices of traditional healers such as faqirs, maulanas, and pandits, among others, were often derogatively referred to as 'folk medicine'.[14] The subordination of Indian

---

[12] Dols, 'Insanity and Its Treatment in Islamic Society': 7.

[13] Weiss, 'Critical Study of Unmada', 2.

[14] Waltraud Ernst, *Mad Tales from the Raj: The European Insane in British India, 1800–1858* (London: Routledge, 1991), 80.

medical traditions continued unabashedly in the context of insanity and its treatment as well. James Wise, the Superintendent of the Dacca asylum, argued:

> Hindoo physicians hold that by the derangements of three humours (air, bile, phlegm) all diseases are produced. They recognise six form of insanity, three being the consequence of alteration in these humours; one of the abnormal combination of the humours; another these result of violent passions, and the last the effects of poison. These alternative depend upon improper food, on cursing the gods, Brahmins, or spiritual teachers on the malignant influence of planets, of eclipse, &c. Insanity, leprosy, pthisis, and all incurable diseases are stated by shastras to be the consequence of sins of a former birth ... The treatment of insanity, according to Hindu medicine is very simple. It consists of cold douches, of cooling sherbets, of the milk of the coconut, and of a carminatives with aperients. Vegetable oils, such as those obtained from almond and violet, are rubbed on the scalp. Shutting the patient up to a dark room is highly recommended; and if he behaves improperly, he is to be 'beaten up with a whip.' In some parts of Bengal frog soup is a favourite remedy for insanity, and among the Feringee—the degenerate descendants of the Portuguese—a live frog fastened on the top of the shaven scalp is reputed to be a sovereign remedy for extracting the morbid heat which causes mania.
>
> The opinions held by the Mahomedan-yunani-physicians regarding insanity are less extravagant and absurd. They teach that madness arises from weakness or disorder of the humours of the brain, and from excess of blood and bile. When the patient is robust, they bleed, prescribe purgatives ... To expel the devil, they use amulets on which verse of Koran was written, charms of various kinds, or they burn a piece of paper under patient's nose, on which certain cabalistic words have been traced.[15]

The subordination of Indian notions of madness is associated with colonialism, racism, and hostility towards dominant healing practices. Their vehement condemnation was often couched in derogatory language and expressed the disgust and insecurities felt by the colonial officials towards Indian Ayurvedic and Unani healing systems, often regarded

[15] Sir James Clark's Enquiry.

as superstitious and out of date. Absurdities such as 'a live frog fastened on the top of the shaven scalp' mirror a vivid imagination on the part of British officials as they typecast and mocked Indian healing cultures.

Not only were the indigenous systems of healing attacked but also shrines where the insane were kept for centuries were relegated as sites of barbarism and cruelty. Some of these shrines had been a safe haven for those who were considered to be a burden by their families. One such famous shrine was that of Shah Daula. The shrine is well-known for the care and custody of microcephalics. It has a long history and was established sometime in the sixteenth century. Nothing much is known about the early years of the shrine but a detailed documented history exists for the past 150 years. M. Miles describes Shah Daula in the following words:

> Shah Daulah was born in the second half of the sixteenth century CE, and served his novitiate as a *pir* (holy man) at Sialkot. He then settled at Gujrat, and is believed to have engaged in extensive building works, charitable deeds, teaching and counselling, the care and company of wild animals, and the performance of miracles. His association with microcephalic *chuas*[16] arose in the miracle department, linked with the animal field. Like other *pirs*, Shah Daulah was expected to treat women for infertility. Following his intercessions, some women produced *chuas*. Here the legends diverge, displaying the efforts of creative minds to involve common logic in their rodentology.[17]

The legendary associations of microcephalics with the shrine underwent various twists and turns. The shrine came under the scrutiny of British government officials who had something that amounted to an obsession with Shah Daula's shrine. From the mid-nineteenth century onwards, the Superintendent's of the lunatic asylum keenly observed and recorded various practices of the shrine. Johnson Wilson noted, 'women stealthily seek the temple, and there pass the night; on awaking next morning they find only a chua beside them; this is supposed to influence conception,

---

[16] *Chua*, that is, literally 'mice' refers to microcephalics because of their smaller head size.

[17] M. Miles, 'Pakistan's Microcephalic *Chuas* of Shah Daulah: Cursed, Clamped or Cherished?', *History of Psychiatry*, vol. 7 (1996): 572.

and re-produce chuas *ad libitum*.[18] These rumours further added more investigations by colonial officials. G. F. W. Ewens remarked, 'Rightly or wrongly, a certain amount of mystery, etc., has always been associated with them. They are usually to be met with wandering about the country, each under the faqir, and their pitiful appearance and condition is undoubtedly used as a means of exciting sympathy.'[19] These discourses evoked pity, neglect, and accusations of artificial deformation of skulls of 'mice' or *chuas* (as microcephalics were commonly referred to) by the dargah patrons. The sites of healing, which provided shelter to the mentally retarded, were denounced as places where mentally ill patients were condemned and brutalized.

Indigenous systems of healing were regarded as 'antiquated' and 'superstitious' especially when compared to 'modern' conceptualizations of madness and its treatment. I have already argued that the asylums were regarded as unpopular. A majority of the people did not have access

[18] J. Wilson Johnston, 'Ethnology of the Chuas of Shawdowla Temple, Goojrat, Punjab', *Indian Medical Gazette*, vol. 1 (1866): 111.

[19] G. F. W. Ewens, 'An Account of the Race of Idiots Found in the Punjab Commonly Known as "Shah Daulah's Mice"', in *Insanity in India: Its Symptoms and Diagnosis: With Reference to the Relation of Crime and Insanity* (Calcutta: Thacker, Spink & co., 1908), 335. There existed an unhealthy obsession on the part of British officials with shrines like that of Shah Daulah's. For more details, see Annual Report on the Lunatic Asylums in the Punjab for 1883. There exists description about the physical appearance and behaviour of the chuas. However, the report concludes that 'no evidence' was found of forcible compression of the microcephalics. Editorial, 'Shah Dowla's Mice', *Indian Medical Gazette*, vol. 19 (1884): 271. The editorial also argues that there is no basis to the theory of forcible moulding of chuas' heads. On the other hand rumours regarding deformation of the chuas' head continue to appear. J. M. Longworth Dames argued chuas' heads were deformed by mothers in order to dedicate their children to the saint in 'Shah Daula's "Rats"', *Man*, vol. 15, (1915): 88–9. Charles Lodge Patch rejected the popular hypothesis of deforming the head. He was medical superintendent of the Punjab Mental Hospital, Lahore, and wrote the article, 'Microcephaly: A Report on "The Shah Daulah's Mice"', *Indian Medical Gazette*, vol. 63 (1928): 297–301. I owe the detailed bibliographic details on 'microcephalics of Shah Daulah' to M. Miles. He generously shared his meticulously annotated chronological bibliography.

to the asylums since large numbers of people were illiterate and could not understand the formal procedure that needed to be followed to secure admission for their near ones. The Indian population had little trust in modern healing mechanisms. In times of distress they relied on traditional ideas of sickness and cure. Historians have discussed how patients very often consulted various healers, and it is generally regarded as 'healer hopping'.[20] Social stigma and class-related anxieties were other significant factors which prevented patients from more frequent use of mental hospitals. Sarah Ann Pinto argues that 'while violence and abuse within the asylum was a source of trauma to patients, the undermining of Indian worldviews, cultures and beliefs further added to their emotional shock'.[21]

The clash between Indian and Western beliefs and practices forced 'natives' to reformulate their ideas on mental and physical sickness in relation to modernity. This resulted in an elevated and holistic understanding of the mind/body relationship by drawing symbology and terminology from Ayurveda, mesmerism, and hypnotism as well as from the newly formulated psychiatric knowledge. Ayurvedic understandings of mental illness were closely tied to the spiritual well-being of human beings. Mental balance and spiritual consciousness were twin sides of the same coin. Ayurvedic practitioners felt an urgent need to reiterate and often reconceptualize basic ideals for healthy mind and body. Pandit Chhavidutt Vaidyaraj in his article 'Mansik Rog Kyun Hota Hain' (what causes mental illness) in the journal *Ayurveda Vigyan* published in 1932 pointed towards the causes and ways by which one can deal with mental illness. He explained:

> What is mind power? The power which allows us to think is called mind power. This helps in concentration and determination ... What is mind?

[20] 'Healer hopping' means the patient's ability or strategy to visit multiple healers or jump from one healer to another. It also refers to a medically pluralistic society where patients have multiple options. For details, see Waltraud Ernst, *Plural Medicine, Traditions and Modernity, 1800–2000* (London: Routledge, 2002), 2.

[21] Sarah Ann Pinto, 'Shackled Bodies, Unchained Minds: Lunatic Asylums in Bombay Presidency, 1793–1921', unpublished doctoral thesis, Victoria University of Wellington, 2017, 5.

This is to clarify that according to Indian context mind and soul are two different things. Soul is eternal, imperishable and free from disorders where mind is regarded perishable. However, the modern medicinal system does not regard mind and body as two different things ... It [soul] is the power which stabilizes life-force in the body and one of its characteristics is knowledge ... As the magnetic energies transmit from one to another metal object similarly the energy which transmits from human body settles into heart and the energy which transmits from mind and soul assembles into brain; and both attempt to maintain the body in their own capacities.[22]

In Indian philosophical traditions, *atman* or soul was regarded as essential along with mind or *manas* for working of the body. The *Caraka Samhita* regarded insanity to be a result of inadequate diet, anger of gods, grief, and fear. The *Caraka Samhita* also pointed out that mental illness can occur due to an unstable state of consciousness, memory, understanding, and mind.

The following sections will elaborate how ancient ideas were reiterated in modern ways. The colonial administration not only neglected Indian ideals of living but also attempted to replace them with modern mechanisms of the state. Asylums should be regarded as intrinsic to colonial governance and a 'tool of empire'. The lunatic asylums not only reflected the desire of colonial officials to physically incapacitate local populations who could pose a 'danger' to the stability of the Raj, but were also a concomitant means to emasculate the mind and body of the colonized. Modernization meant bringing in modern technologies, institutions, and infrastructure to replace traditional ways of life. Modern India witnessed socio-religious reforms that attempted the eradication of social and religious evils such as sati, endeavoured to popularize widow remarriage, and raised the age of consent.[23] Medicine also underwent a phase of reform and revival which was characteristically different from other socio-religious reforms. What needs to be kept in mind is that when faced with rapid changes, traditional mental healing practices focused

---

[22] Pandit Chhavidutt Vaidyaraj, 'Mansik Rog Kyun Hota Hain' (What Causes Mental Illness), *Ayurveda Vigyan*, part 2 (February 1932): 287, 289–90.

[23] Kenneth Jones, *Socio-Religious Reform Movements in British India* (Albany: State University of New York Press, 1992).

on select areas that were thought to be destabilizing their social order. Spiritual writings on healing the mind witnessed a sudden upsurge. Such writings on mental healing often borrowed Western terminology and techniques to appeal to the newly emergent middle class. Sexual anxieties arising due to communal tensions and fears of degeneration proliferated. Gender was a central marker in the medical and socio-cultural constructions of insanity and associated anxieties.

Psychotherapy and Its Discontents

Psychotherapy is a quintessentially Western concept. It implies a clinical setting where the paid psychologists or psychiatrist attempts to provide therapy usually through counselling and less frequently through medication. This does not imply that psychotherapy cannot be provided in traditional societies. Recent scholarship, in fact, points to the efficacy of psychotherapy by locally available healers as it helps patients to relate their problems and issues closely.[24] The reinterpretation of Western concepts and their co-option with Indian notions of sickness and cure were unique and significant. The circulation of knowledge occurred at multiple levels. The popular and elite notions were reconceptualized in the light of Western knowledge. This could be simply because of the competition in the medical markets as well as acculturation over time which cannot be discounted easily.

Durgashankar Nagar's book *Prana Chikitsa (Psycho-Therapy—It's Doctrine and Practice)*[25] emphasized the centrality of mind/body healing

---

[24] Medical anthropologists, psychologists, and psychiatrists have emphasized on the efficacy of healing traditions to treat psychological problems. It has also been argued that mental health care system should include centres of faith as they promote spiritual and psychological recovery for the patients and their caregivers. For details, see Murphy Halliburton, *Mudpacks and Prozac: Experiencing Ayurvedic, Biomedical and Religious Healing* (California: Left Coast Press, 2009); Shubha Ranganathan, 'Healing Temples, the Anti-Superstition Discourse and Global Mental Health: Some Questions from Mahanubhav Temples in India', *South Asia: Journal of South Asian Studies*, vol. 37, no. 4 (2014): 625–39.

[25] Durgashankar Nagar, *Prana Chikitsa (Psycho-Therapy—It's Doctrine and Practice)* (Lucknow: Adhyaksha Ganga Fine Art Press, 1931).

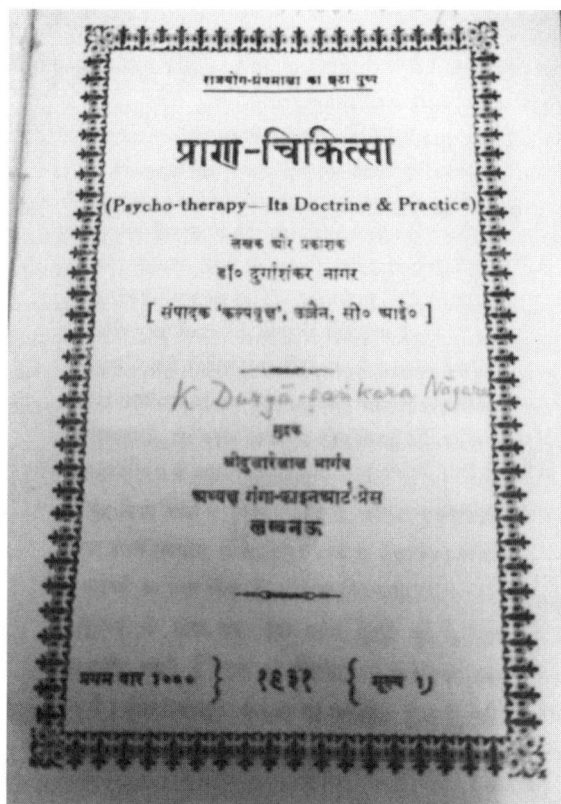

Figure 5.1   Page from *Prana Chikitsa*
Source: British Library, UK.

and its implication of mental, psychical, and physical healing (Figure 5.1). The word *prana* can be understood variously as 'life', 'soul', 'spirit', 'breath', and 'vitality'. The translation of *Prana Chikitsa* here may be regarded as 'life's cure' since *chikitsa* means cure and the broader meaning of the term 'prana' can be interpreted as life. Nagar's book was published in Lucknow in 1931. He is addressed as 'doctor' though it is unknown whether he had any medical degree or not. Rather, the practice of using the medical title of 'doctor' for himself can be contextualized as an attempt to widen the popularity of his book, while authenticating its Western medical connections, among the growing middle class. His translation, use, and equation of the word 'prana' to the English word 'psychotherapy' can also be construed as an attempt to reach a more scientifically inclined society. Modern ideas had a wide appeal and self-fashioning should also be understood as a technique of marketing.

Prana Chikitsa equated life's element to the mesmerisitic concept of 'magnetism' and also derived legitimacy from yogic and tantric ancient Indian traditions. The author argued:

> People who theorize Mesmerism says its stays in body in pulse only in form of water and other subtle substances [*sic*]. It is found in abundance only in forehead and spinal cord. We have its detailed description in our Tantra system. Vitality exists only in body. Its origin is in sex body and in similar way in subtle substance of pulses. In spinal cord it is found mainly in form of substance but it mainly exists above forehead and its main existence is in heart only. Its velocity is continuous on both places and its flow is continuous through both nostrils which are called sun and the moon.[26]

Franz Mesmer developed a technique called 'mesmerism' or 'magnetism' which was based on the principle that all living or non-living beings have energy or what he called 'animal magnetism'. This magnetic energy can be channelized in order to cure various diseases. He strongly believed that diseases are caused due to imbalances in this magnetic fluid. Mesmer initially used magnets to cure his patients but later shifted to massages and passes from hand to heal various illnesses. Mesmerism was extremely popular in eighteenth-century France. Robert Darnton points out that 'mesmerism was debated in the academies, salons, and cafes. It was investigated by the police, patronized by the queen, ridiculed several times on the stage, burlesqued in popular songs, doggerels, and cartoons, practiced in a network of masonic-like secret societies, and publicized by a flood of pamphlets and books'.[27] In spite of this initial fervour, mesmerism lost its popularity. Nonetheless, it continued to be sporadically evoked in popular imaginings and resurfaced in several parts of the globe during the nineteenth and twentieth centuries in several spiritualistic, hypnotic, and psychotherapeutic movements. 'Tantrism' is considered a protean term defining Indian traditions. These traditions, claims Andrea

---

[26] Nagar, *Prana Chikitsa*, 4.

[27] Robert Darnton, *Mesmerism and the End of the Enlightenment in France* (Cambridge: Harvard University Press, 1968), 40–1.

Padoux, constitute 'the ideological aspect of the Tantric vision', which is 'the cosmos as permeated by power (or powers), a vision wherein energy (*sakti*) is both cosmic and human and where microcosm and macrocosm correspond and interact'.[28]

John Warne Monroe argues that 'a new understanding of the beyond' was part of innovative religious beliefs and practices associated with mesmerism from the 1850s onwards. During the period, heterodoxy surfaced in novel forms as a common feature of middle-class urban life.[29] Nagar's attempts of fusing mesmerism with Tantrism should be located within these globalized movements which rekindled spirituality and amalgamated it with scientific repertoire to gain legitimacy. However, he only makes indirect references to Tantric ideas. He did not delve into the concept of sakti or power in detail. He rather uses a more Westernized notion of 'magnetic' energy found in human beings. His selections of ideas and practices were more Western than Indian which is remarkable as it mirrors his attempts to gain legitimacy from both sides.

The colonial period witnessed enormous changes that included inventions and introductions of modern-day technologies such as medical procedures that were often invasive but life-saving. Electricity, railways, telephones, typewriters, and sewing machines are a few other examples of life-transforming experiences. Historians have delineated experiences of people from different strata of society when faced with the new world. New psychological intervention was also one such invention. Freudian ideas gained enormous popularity in Bengal. India, in fact, had one of the earliest departments of psychology (see Chapter 1). Nonetheless, there has been no research so far on the percolation of these ideas among the lay people. Nagar's book provides this unique opportunity to fathom how these concepts were perceived in the Indo-Gangetic belt at the time.

Psychology and religion have shared a long and complicated relationship. Psychiatry and psychology borrowed their underlying

---

[28] Andre Padoux, 'What Do We Mean by Tantrism', in *The Roots of Tantra*, edited by Katherine Anne Harper and Robert L. Brown (New York: State University of New York Press, 2002), 19. For more details, see David Gordon White, *Sinister Yogis* (Chicago: University of Chicago Press, 2009).

[29] John Warne Monroe, *Laboratories of Faith: Mesmerism, Spiritism and Occultism in Modern France* (London: Cornell University Press, 2008), 3.

healing concepts from religion. Dinesh Bhugra emphasizes that 'one may argue that psychiatry took over from religion and created its own high church and in extraordinary developments, unlike religion, locked people away in a physical space.'[30] When religion lost its monopoly over healing, it was forced to reinvent itself due to unprecedented modernization. Therefore, the reinforcement of physical cultures went hand in hand with reformulations of mental healing and its sub-cultures in colonial India.

Nagar remarked that 'man has hidden power that is called vim power or vital force which is also termed as magnetism. Regulating that basic element of life by attracting it is what is discussed in the spiritual teaching method.'[31] His belief in a hidden power corresponds to ancient yogic traditions of evoking and mastering the mind to channelize energy but reference to words such as 'vim' and 'magnetism' mirror modern influences and the need to recast variegated practices. Disturbance in vim can cause diseases and especially diseases of the pulse and nerve can be cured by regulation of vital force or vim. He claimed to heal diseases ranging from hysteria, sleeplessness, constipation, diarrhoea, impotence, premature ejaculation, palpitation, sweating, and indigestion. These assertions were based on the power of the mind. He argued, 'The mind resides in every bit of the human body. This is not all, the mind is present in all objects in the world, it resides in all of the world, or is omnipresent. The miracles that are visible in the world, they are all by the mind. Mind is the only conscious force.'[32] This urgent need to situate and use every possible technique ranging from ancient wisdom to newer ideas of magnetism were attempts to place the 'mind' at the centre of curing a number of illnesses. The nationalist struggle and its responses to colonial domination reflect the desire of not only building physical strength but also of training the mind to heal visible and invisible ailments. There was also a trend to invent cures which would act like a 'panacea' for every sickness known to mankind. Ayurvedic practitioners, who were facing competition from Western medical paraphernalia, attempted miraculous cures

---

[30] Dinesh Bhugra (ed.), *Psychiatry and Religion: Context, Consensus and Controversies* (London: Routledge. 1996), 230.

[31] Nagar, *Prana Chikitsa*, 9.

[32] Nagar, *Prana Chikitsa*, 27.

with less invasive techniques and prescriptions of a supposed panacea in order to draw people from different walk of lives.

Psychics or traditional healers have been known for their ability to heal sickness related to the mind and body by providing an outlet to people suffering from depression or anxiety. Their ability to lend a patient ear to those who were in distress and forge bonds based on their understanding of local and communal problems helped them act as psychotherapists for thousands of years. Nagar in his book attempted to re-enact the psychiatric/psychic amalgam. He pointed out:

> The first thing that a mental healer should do is to listen to the description of the patient from start to end, very carefully, not a single part should be missed. The patient feels very re-assured by it. It does not matter if it takes time. In other diseases, there is not much need for so much questioning and discussion, but in mental (psychoneurosis) diseases, it is important to know the entire description. Along with that, the patient's life character, daily life should be known. Other than that it should be known whether the disease was induced from—school life, mother, father, brother, sister, friends, and other relatives, etc, and other life matters should be carefully studied. The patients' religious and moral beliefs, social life, and the aims of his/her life, etc, all should be known. It is from these words of the patient that one gets to know the patients' inner mind.[33]

It is interesting to note that Nagar himself used the English term 'psychiatrist' which he equates with mental healer (himself). His frequent references to medical jargon such as 'psychoneurosis', 'psychosis', 'psychotherapy', 'psychoanalysis', and 'will power', only to name a few, reflect further attempts at amalgamating psychiatric repertoire written in English with Hindi medical vocabulary. Vernacularization of Western psychiatrist knowledge often utilized English words but meanings sometimes changed depending on the context or usage. Psychoneurosis here refers to neurosis which meant emotional conflicts faced by patients that were causing his/her behavioural problems. Moreover, references to how imperative it was to know the patient's history, such as 'religious and moral beliefs, social life and the aims of his/her life', point towards

[33] Nagar, *Prana Chikitsa*, 19.

incorporation of Eastern and Western practices of mind sciences. The preceding description resonates with the Freudian method of delving into the unconscious mind. The things that were missing are a couch and the technique. The techniques used to heal were derived from the mesmerist traditions. According to Nagar, hands should be used to massage the lower abdomen or any part which needs to be cleansed. There are two types of forces in nature. One is positive and the other negative. Similarly, a human body can be made strong by cleansing the body of negativity and filling it with positive energy. He further points out that 'the hands should massage downwards from head to toe and release those rapidly to throw away the bad energy accumulated in the palms.'[34]

Mesmer believed that sickness was a consequence of blocking the flow of fluid through the body. The massaging of the body supposedly helped in healing and restoring health.[35] In spite of continuous reference to magnetism and magnetic therapy, Nagar did not refer to the use of magnets in his treatment. Instead, he emphasized the role of vim power or vital force which he also termed as magnetism. He also believed in self-treatment. He explained a technique by which one can cure one's illnesses.

> I am the soul, I am the ocean of all strength. From my self-will, all the nerves of my body are getting nutrient and strength. I do not require any substance. From today I am leaving behind the attraction of addictive substances. I am the form of consciousness. Form of strength. I am above everyone.[36]

It is difficult to fathom the popularity of Nagar's work. His theories were empowering to those who were depressed or suffering from other mental diseases. The belief in 'self-will', 'strength', and 'consciousness' was regarded as significant to cure one's sickness. His strategies of mental healing had vital techniques, self-endorsing terminology, and miraculous claims of curing to incurable diseases. These conjectures when

[34] Nagar, *Prana Chikitsa*, 102.

[35] For more details, see Adam Crabtree, *From Mesmer to Freud: Magnetic Sleep and the Roots of Psychological Healing* (New Haven: Yale University Press, 1993).

[36] Nagar, *Prana Chikitsa*, 60.

understood in the climate of unparalleled globalized, nationalized, and localized changes were a recipe for a powerful text. Mechanization of human life was a worldwide phenomenon, which also has parallels with national emaciation and degenerative paranoia. Further, the lack of infrastructure related to modern psychiatry available to people living in smaller towns should be situated as contexts in which the book was written and ideas of 'self-cure' were published and peddled.

By the third decade of the twentieth century, psychotherapy was at its zenith and was extremely popular throughout the globe. Nagar's book, written during the same period, shows its far-reaching impact. Nagar's *Prana Chikitsa*, although outmoded since he does not directly refer to either Freud or his contemporaries, was based on the use, reinvention, and jumbling up of ideas from contemporary Western medical ideas as well as ancient Indian and mesmeric notions and techniques. Mostly, Nagar considered himself to be a psychotherapist, although sometimes a psychiatrist. Nonetheless, he identified himself more as a psychotherapist as the book *Prana Chikitsa* was simultaneously named as 'psychotherapy'.

The basic difference between psychotherapy and psychiatry is inherently based on the fact that the former is based on the 'talking cure' and the latter attempts to deal with more severe cases with the intervention of medication. There has been intense competition between the two practices wherein psychotherapy is mostly regarded to be subordinate to psychiatry. Psychotherapy is based on psychology, which still struggles to gain acceptance as a 'science'. Psychiatry, on the other hand, is considered to be integral to medical science. Nonetheless, Nagar claimed the superiority of a psychotherapist over a psychiatrist:

> Psychiatric treatment has capacity to recognize diseases with much ease. Medical knowledge explains how pain, sufferings and symptoms in different components of body are termed with different names. But we have innumerable list of diseases which are still difficult to be diagnosed. And it also takes longer time to diagnose the disease until right medicine actually reaches the body. There is also fear of side effects in such cases. This is not expected out of those people who are psychotherapist. Psychotherapy only focuses on life force driving organs as heart, digestive organs, liver, kidney, spinal cord, and organs involved in blood circulation. It does not distinguish on basis of names but attempts to recognize it in relation to

life force driving organs. This tries to cure disease by using natural consciousness, will power, soul power and knowingness to root out its basic
cause.[37]

He accepted the superiority of medical knowledge but maintained his
pre-eminence by focusing on what he called life force. Side effects of psychiatric medicine are highlighted, whereas unknown diseases are claimed
to be cured by focusing on inner energies. 'Natural consciousness', 'will
power', and 'soul power' were highly individualized concepts which were
more spiritual than religious. Nagar's reference to religion was loose and
also syncretized, which allowed wider access of his therapies.

His mental healing theory explained the Western modern notions
about suppressed sexuality and altered it. He argued:

> Another method is to reignite the desires in the mind, and convert them
> into sexual yearning. Then by paying respect to the life-force devoid body
> of the person we should reignite the dying flame by recharging the hor-
> monal activity through outside energy ... Many psychological problems
> are caused due to ethereal matter in the brain. They are cured by the
> magnetic therapy. It is just like a numb body gets rejuvenated and it also
> revitalizes the mental and physiological energy in the body ... A person
> who does not pay attention to the sexual needs of the body and gets irri-
> tated over trivial matters, aggravated, feels pressurised and nervous in
> dealing with small problems, anxiety, affects not only itself, but also badly
> injures the other person giving rise to new diseases.[38]

These ideas were in stark contrast to the more puritanical Hindu trends
that were widely accepted during the period. Men and women were
expected to maintain total self-control and advised only to utilize sexual
energies for the purpose of reproduction. It can be argued that Nagar
was much ahead of his times since he recognized the need to unleash
suppressed sexual desires. His belief in rationality had its own limits,
however. In his book, he describes detailed ways in which the healer
should capture ghosts. He believed that the spirit was capable of harm-
ing humans. But there are methods by which the spirits can be dealt

[37] Nagar, *Prana Chikitsa*, 8.
[38] Nagar, *Prana Chikitsa*, 11–12.

with. He narrates an array of equipment such as *tabeez* (amulet), astrological mirror, rings, and '[using] camphor balls and putting it in a bronze metal plate and mixing cow-ghee with it should apply it on the windows of the house to ward off any bad spirits from entering.'[39] The belief in magnetic, magical, tantric, and psychic traditions mirrors the anxieties of the self in a colonial milieu. There existed a thin line between quackery and professionalized medicine as far the history of science and medicine is concerned while 'science' and 'religion' were often blurred categories. The development of 'science' from pseudo-sciences has to be recognized to comprehend the borrowing of ideas, techniques, and concepts of psychiatry and psychology from a number of spiritual practices. Robert Darnton highlights that mesmerism was not only considered fashionable but it was also regarded as 'scientific' in eighteenth-century France. *Prana Chitiktsa* borrowed from mesmerism or psychotherapy derived from yogic/tantric/vedic ideas, which cannot be clearly distinguished. What separates them is the fact that *Prana Chitiktsa* changed the meaning of psychotherapy by emphasizing on the significance of mind/body healing practices.

Nagar's book *Prana Chikitsa* reflects the packing together of ancient and modern, Eastern and Western, and popular and elite traditions which gave birth to new hybrid mental healing practices. Nile Green argues that historians have so far failed to recognize the fact that Indian mysticism had an underlying political dimension to the physical and psychological acts of conditioning and control in Indian meditation systems.[40] In a similar vein, the emergence of mind sciences, which broadly included the rise of psychiatry and psychology, and their stepchild, psychic and related ubiquitous psychological healing practices in the Indian medical tradition, mirror the needs of time.[41]

[39] Nagar, *Prana Chikitsa*, 90.

[40] Nile Green, 'Breathing in India, c. 1890', *Modern Asian Studies*, vol. 42, no. 2/3 (March–May 2008): 293.

[41] For more details, see Heather Wolfram, *The Stepchildren of Science, Psychical Research and Parapsychology in Germany, c. 1870–1939* (Amsterdam: Rodopi, 2009); Andreas Sommer, 'Psychical Research in the History and Philosophy of Science: An Introduction and Review', *Studies in History and Philosophy of Biological and Biomedical Sciences*, vol. 48 (2014): 38–45.

Psycho-sexual Health and Nationalist Anxieties

Semen was considered to be the most essential bodily element and its conservation was regarded as crucial to the maintenance of a healthy mind and body. The nationalist anxieties projected 'celibacy' as the only possible cure to save the degenerate 'Hindu' nation. It was believed that masturbation ruined the lives of the Hindu youth and created a degenerate Hindu nation. As Charu Gupta argues, 'Brahmacharya thus became a building block for claims to social and political power, cultural identity and a "scientific" way of life.'[42] The psychosexual medical literature of the period mourned the degeneration of the Hindu nation. It was vehemently argued that morally weak men lacked the mental strength to keep themselves away from modern vices and thereby they lost their mental and bodily health. Western discourses on masturbation and madness were not directly linked to each other in the Hindi medical literature. However, anxieties surrounding masturbation or *hasthmaithun*, loss of semen, and manliness were related to one's mental inability to control such 'self-depraving' urges.

The Western and Eastern notions of well-being were integrated and key categories of psychosexual pathologies emerged in late nineteenth- and early twentieth-century Indian medical systems. Ayurvedic and Unani medical traditions considered semen to be the essence of life.[43] Its preservation was considered quintessential for the conservation of the life element. The modern period witnessed the reigniting of these ideas in a more aggressive manner. The fears of degeneration were widespread due to the creation of the Muslim as the 'Other'. Rumours regarding the increase in the Muslim population and a concomitant decline in the Hindu population led to anxieties around manliness. Heightened communal tensions, electoral politics, and a scramble for jobs need to be contextualized in order to understand the desperate

[42] Charu Gupta, *Sexuality, Obscenity, Community: Women, Muslims and the Hindu Public in Colonial India* (New York: Palgrave, 2002), 69.

[43] For more details, see Kenneth G. Zysk, 'Potency Therapy in Classical Indian Medicine', *Asian Medicine*, vol. 1, no. 1 (2005): 101–118; Anna Winterbottom and Facil Tesfaye, eds, *Histories of Medicine and Healing in the Indian Ocean World*, vol. 1 (London: Palgrave Macmillan, 2016).

need for 'self-preservation'.[44] Numerous tracts were written on the significance of *brahmcharya* or celibacy. Pandit Ganeshdutt Indra in his treatise *Swapnadosh Vigyan* or *The Science of Nocturnal Emissions*[45] used a Sanskrit phrase to delineate the significance of brahmcharya as follows:

Brahmacharyan tamsa deva mrityumupadhananth[46]

Celibacy was considered the ideal way to overcome death as used by the gods. In other words, semen is the sacred nectar. The one who contains this nectar attains immortality.[47] He further argued 'according to the *Dharmashastra* ... young men should not even spend solitary time with their mother. Even if such occasion arises, when one has to speak to a woman, they should talk to the lady softly and decently and by not looking directly at her.'[48] These manuals were didactic in nature and drew legitimacy by evoking vedic and shastric literature.

Colonialism and nationalism shared an intricate relationship with masculinity. Mrinalini Sihna argues that the dynamism between colonial and nationalistic politics can best be understood through the logic of colonial masculinity. She asserts, 'for colonial masculinity points towards the multiple axes along which power was exercised in colonial India: among or within the colonisers and the colonised as well as between colonisers and colonised'.[49] Through the widespread use of chastizing

---

[44] Gupta, *Sexuality, Obscenity and Community*, 4. For a discussion on communalism, see Vasudha Dalmia, *The Nationalisation of Hindu Traditions: Bharatendu Harischandra and Nineteenth-Century Banaras* (Oxford University Press: Delhi, 1997); Christophe Jaffrelot, *The Hindu Nationalist Movement and Indian Politics: 1925 to the 1990s* (London: Hurst & Company, 1996); and Francis Robinson, *Separatism among Indian Muslims: The Politics of the UP Muslims, 1860–1923* (Delhi: Oxford University Press, 1993).

[45] Pandit Ganeshdutt Indra, *Swapnadosh Vigyan* (Kashi: Kailashnath Bhargav 'Amar', 1949).

[46] Translated, it means 'Through celibacy, the gods conquer death'. Indra, *Swapnadosh Vigyan*, 7.

[47] Indra, *Swapnadosh* Vigyan, 7.

[48] Indra, *Swapnadosh Vigyan*, 75.

[49] Mrinalini Sinha. *Colonial Masculinity: The 'Manly Englishman' and the 'Effeminate Bengali' in the Late Nineteenth Century* (New York: Manchester University Press, 1995), 1.

literature, there was a serious attempt to create hyper-masculine Hindu men. These identities contested and clashed and played a significant role in redefining gender, class, and caste. Not only were the bodies made a site of introspection but this peddled medical literature blamed 'weak minds' for corrupting the self and society. The purpose of these pamphlets and articles was to generate fears in the bodies and minds of the youth. Moral rhetoric suffused with sickness and death were used to deter men who had fallen prey to modernity.

Another pamphlet entitled *Naujawan Kyun Maarey Jaate Hain* noted:

> These days young men and adults are dying due of tuberculosis, heart diseases, mental illness and other illnesses leaving their loved one in pain. And this is because, they have wasted youth and weakened their body by self abusing. The consequence of this self abuse is it weakens the strength of nerves and muscles, which results in epilepsy, shivering of hands and paralysis. Many lose their senses and sanity and end up in the lunatic asylum. The self abuse is widespread in our society is actually worse than suicide.[50]

It further stated,

> I am explaining all this so that I can save you from the path of destruction, and so that young men do not die before time. If one rubs his penis then blood flow increases in the region, which leads to weakness and consequently other body parts become deficient of blood circulation. Nerves of penis are connected to the spinal cord and brain.[51]

By connecting the mind to the body an attempt was made to generate self-loathing among those individuals who considered their own interests over the welfare of the nation. The power of the mind and its relationship to the body was put on centre stage by nationalists who widened the concept of self-abuse. Control over one's self became central to one's ability to serve the country. Joseph Alter describes that 'it is a common belief among Hindus that the essence of life is contained in semen ...

---

[50] Anonymous, *Naujawan Kyun Maarey Jaate Hain* (Why young men die?) (Lahore: Anglo-Sanskrit Press Lahore, n.d.), 28.

[51] Anonymous, *Naujawan Kyun Maarey Jaate Hain*, 13.

Not only do they regard semen as the quintessential fluid of life, they also regard it as the very cornerstone of their somatic enterprise. It is the source of all strength, all energy, all knowledge, all skill.[52] Alter is here discussing the significance of the belief of brahmcharya in the Hindu *akharas* (gymnasiums). The wrestler's way of life required complete abstinence from any sort of sexual activity.

Graeco-Roman thought also regarded semen as the single most essential fluid. Mels Van Driel remarks:

> While Hippocrates assigned a more or less equal role to the man and the woman, Aristotle took a different view. Of course he could not help admitting some female input and so argued that woman's sole contribution was to provide what he called *catamenia*. This was residual menstrual blood that constituted transformed matter and could basically produce nothing until the man added his seed. The drawings of Leonardo da Vinci (1452–1519) show his brilliant mind still clinging to the idea that seminal fluid came straight from the brain. Leonardo drew two ducts in the penis, one for the passage of urine and one for seminal fluid. The white seminal fluid came like mother's milk directly from the backbone.[53]

Superiority of male over female was established by pointing out that the female's role in reproduction was much lesser than man's. From the Middle Ages, it was also ascertained that the seminal fluid came from the brain. These ideas were internalized by ideologues in twentieth-century India. The wastage of semen emerged as a pandemic in eighteenth-century Europe. The modern discourse on masturbation and its amalgamation into psychiatric knowledge was accepted as something sacrosanct up till the beginning of the twentieth century. Madness, masturbation, and the so-called elements of the brain have a complicated history which travelled across the globe taking mythic forms, giving rise to imaginary diseases and condemning the idea of self-love.

---

[52] Joseph S. Alter, *The Wrestler's Body: Identity and Ideology in North India* (Berkeley: University of California Press, 1992), 108.

[53] Mels Van Driel, *Manhood: The Rise and Fall of the Penis* (London: Reaktion Books, 2009), 13.

Thomas Laqueur argues that sometime between 1708 and 1716—'in or around 1712'—the then anonymous author of a short tract with a long title not only named but actually invented a new disease and a new 'highly specific, thoroughly modern, and nearly universal engine for generating guilt, shame and anxiety'.[54] He is here referring to the birth of the modern disease of masturbation. Michel Foucault also later pointed out that 'masturbation becomes the cause, the universal causality of every illness'.[55] In the context of India, masturbation became a disease 'par excellence' by the last decades of nineteenth century. Ishita Pande regards that along with other pathologies of the empire, masturbation should be understood as 'a story of the entwinement of politics and medicine, power and knowledge, in the age of empire'.[56]

The Western concept of 'self-abuse' constituted discourses around masturbation, insanity, and impotency. 'Self-abuse' as an idea essentially meant solitary sex. Whereas in the Indian context the notion of 'self-abuse' included any sort of sexual activity which intended pleasure for the sake of sexual gratification. The Hindi pamphlet *Swapnadosh Vigyan* has an interesting conversation between a vaidya and his patient. The patient asked how many times and when one should have sex with a woman.

Vaidya: Once in two years.
Person: If someone cannot control for that long?
Vaidya: Once in a year then.
Person: If someone cannot wait for that long?
Vaidya: One should have once in six months.
Person: If he can't wait for six months then?
Vaidya: He can have sexual intercourse once in three months.
Person: How much time less than that?
Vaidya: Once in a month.
Person: Less than that?
Vaidya: Once in fifteen days.

[54] Thomas W. Laqueur, *Solitary Sex: A Cultural History of Masturbation* (New York: Zone Books, 2003).

[55] Michel Foucault, *Abnormal: Lectures at the College de France 1974–75*, translated by Graham Burchell (New Delhi: Navayana, 2010), 241.

[56] Ishita Pande, *Medicine, Race and Liberalism in British Bengal: Symptoms of Empire* (London: Routledge), 16.

Person: Less than that?

Vaidya (taking a deep breath):   Once in a week.

Person: Less than that?

Vaidya (irritated):   One can do it twice in a week but cannot remain
healthy and strong.

Person: Less than that?

Vaidya (angrily):   Less than that, whenever he wishes to and he should
get his pyre ready.[57]

Control over the self could only be mastered through regulation of
sexual activity. The images evoked were not of monstrosity or criminality but rather of debilitating, sickly pale men who symbolized a 'dying
Hindu race'. The decline of the mental and moral make-up of youth
was regarded as a significant cause of widespread mortality, child marriage, and other social evils. Nocturnal emission, masturbation, and anal
sex were resulting in the degeneration of society and this was because
of widespread modern vices. Kavi Harnamdas in his pamphlet *Yovan
Raksha* (The protection of youth) (Figure 5.2) asserted that 'youth
get addicted to the vices which results in destruction of their health.
Overindulgences in food, sexual transgressions, watching cinema late at
night, reading romantic novels along with bad company leads to the loss
of life element i.e. semen at an early age'.[58] The advent of modern life
along with increased urbanism was seen as a threat to the moral character of men and women. Changing food values, modern entertainment,
and cheaply available print were regarded as considerable moral threats
destabilizing traditional lifestyle.

While discussing the rise of psychiatric knowledge in Bengali, Amit
Ranjan Basu argues that 'the psychiatric discourse transformed sexuality by bringing in western scientific concept, and created an order of
sexual governance mediated through this knowledge'.[59] Masturbation
in early modern South Asia was discussed in erotological and medical

[57] Indra, *Swapnadosh Vigyan*, 60.

[58] Kavi Harnamdas, *Yovan Raksha* (Lahore: n.p., 1936), 2.

[59] Amit Ranjan Basu, 'Emergence of a Marginal Science in a Colonial City:
Reading Psychiatry in Bengali Periodicals', *The Indian Economic and Social
History Review*, vol. 41, no. 2, (2004): 137.

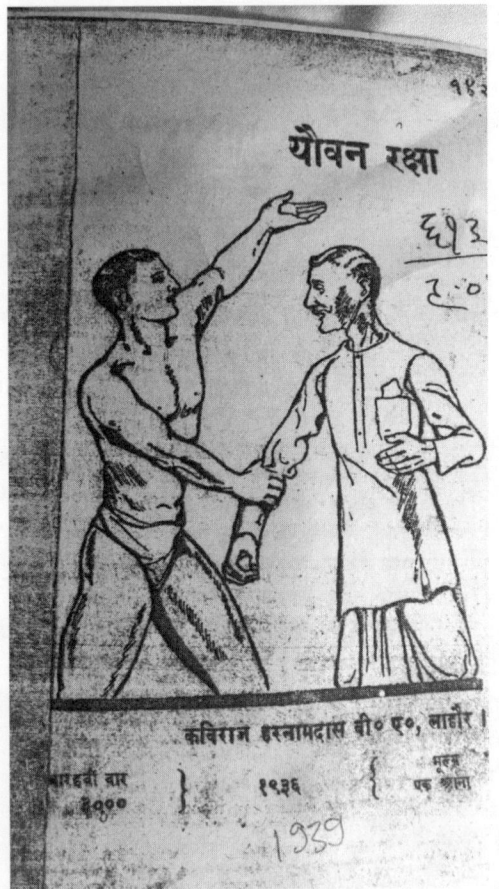

Figure 5.2 First page from *Yovan Raksha*
Source: Hindi Nagari Pracharani Sabha, Collection.

manuals. There is a limited amount of secondary information on the subject.[60] By the latter half of the nineteenth century the physical perils of masturbation were delved into in detail, while the mental dangers of solitary sex were discussed obliquely in Hindi medical literature.

[60] For discussion on medical manuals, see Seema Alavi, *Islam and Healing: Loss and Recovery of an Indo-Muslim Medical Tradition, 1600–1900* (Palgrave Macmillan, 2008); Zysk, 'Potency Therapy in Classical Indian Medicine'.

Unlike Nagar and others who emphasized that utilization of sexual energies was essential for a healthy body and mind, popular Hindi medical literature was influenced by the puritanical elements that had become palpable and aggressive with heightened communal tensions during the period.

Projit Bihari Mukharji points out that Bengali newspapers elaborately discussed advertisements of *dhatu dourbalya*.[61] He quotes Dr Chattopadhyay, who was an authority on the subject, highlighting that 'dhatu loss usually meant losing semen'.[62] He further points out that Chattopadhyay listed a total of 23 'physical' and 14 'mental' symptoms of dhatu dourbalya. The physical symptoms included sunken eyes, roughness of skin, and balding, while mental symptoms often ranged from disorganized thinking and sighing to cowardliness and sleeplessness.[63] Mukharji regards dhatu dourbalya as 'a rhizoid reality composed of numerous shifting names, designation and anxieties'.[64]

Dhatu dourbalya was a Bengali variant of anxieties related to issues around loss of masculinity and nationhood. The Indo-Gangetic belt with increased communal tension witnessed a surge of Hindi medical literature on loss of masculinity.[65] These writings tied loss of physical strength with mental ability. Failure to control sexual urges depended on mental strength, and a 'man' was one who was capable of 'maintaining manly vigour, intelligence, wealth, moral behaviour and courage',[66] whereby he was required to defend community and nation. These fears of degeneration should be connected to what Ashis Nandy has described as 'psychological resistance against colonialism'.[67] These texts reiterate

---

[61] Projit Bihari Mukharji, *Nationalizing the Body: The Medical Market, Print and Daktari Medicine* (London: Anthem Press, 2011), 217. The definition for the term is provided in pages 217 and 218.

[62] Mukharji, *Nationalizing the Body*, 217.

[63] Mukharji, *Nationalizing the Body*, 220.

[64] Mukharji, *Nationalizing the Body*, 247.

[65] The culturally bound syndrome or *dhat* syndrome continues to appear in contemporary psychiatric writing. For details, see, Mukharji, *Nationalizing the Body*, 215–17.

[66] Indra, *Swapnadosh Vigyan*, 41.

[67] Asish, Nandy, *The Intimate Enemy: Loss and Recovery of Self under Colonialism* (Delhi, Oxford University Press, 1983), 12.

feelings of self-hatred, disciplining, and desires to take back control from the oppressors. There is little doubt that in doing so, nationalistic thought went too far from the path of so-called self-recovery. Sexual desire and associated pleasures became taboos and sin. Self-indulgent behaviour was equated with moral delinquency. Thus, preservation of the self was regarded as an exclusive weapon to fight against communal, capitalist, and colonial onslaught.

The most important figure whose 'experiments with the truth' led him to the path of complete self-control was Mohandas Karamchand Gandhi. It should not be mistakenly assumed, however, that semen loss and its links to the loss of manliness resulted entirely from Gandhi's puritanical world view. Rather, these views were part and parcel of the world in which Gandhi evolved and became the Mahatma. Nonetheless, it can be vehemently argued that Gandhi's ideas were idolized and reached the masses with far-reaching consequences. Dreams and the unconscious also became subjects of enquiry. Pandit Ganeshdutt Indra remarked:

> A man with nocturnal emissions always has polluted thoughts. One who has pure thoughts will not face this illness. This sickness is related to dreams, and dreams are 66% linked to the mind. A person can be analysed through his dreams. These kinds of thoughts when fed to your mind gets reflected in your dreams. The power of the mind is a great power, and it is difficult to access it. Therefore, Veda gives ways to maintain a healthy and unpolluted mind.[68]

Gandhi argued that 'it is impossible for unhealthy people to win *swaraj* [self-rule]'.[69] Self-preservation was the key to self-rule.

Masturbation was supposed to be loss of self-control and submission to the most primitive urges of mankind. Onanism emerged as a monstrous act which had pathological links to madness, homosexuality, and criminality. The Indian story translates loss of self-control as loss of self-rule. Ganeshdutt Indra remarked, 'The rubbing, shaking, holding and touching [of] genitals is called "Hastamaithun" or Masturbation. This sexual act has destroyed our country. This sexual practice causes

[68]   Indra, *Swapnadosh Vigyan*, 41.

[69]   Joseph S. Alter, *Gandhi's Body: Sex, Diet, and the Politics of Nationalism* (Philadelphia: University of Pennsylvania Press, 2000), 3.

incurable diseases. Mental hospitals have a number of patients with a history of masturbation.'[70] He also stated, 'Anal sex also causes masturbation. Anal sex is called same sex love and *laundebazi*. People who practice anal sex have pale faces, weak bodies and suffer from mental retardation. Men who indulge in anal sex suffer from number of genital diseases. It is an unnatural act.'[71] There was a serious attempt to define conjugal love, and it was believed that by practising marital hygiene one can not only achieve the desired sex of a child, but also can reproduce superior racial stock. Therefore, masturbation and madness were acts of desecration of the self and society. Chastity and celibacy were the only cures for a dying race. The pandemic of masturbation and madness had very different trajectories in the Eastern and the Western contexts. Nonetheless, there exists striking resemblances as these paths coincided and led to the emergence of a pseudo-science of sexuality in the modern world.[72] The firm belief was that by controlling and regulating desires of the mind and body a 'superior race' could emerge, which was necessary for the survival of communities and nation states.

Hysteria or *Yoshapasmar*

The twentieth century in colonial India witnessed the streamlining of sexual politics related to the moral and domestic arena, wherein men and women were given set roles.[73] Medical ideas, like any other, reflect

---

[70] Indra, *Swapnadosh Vigyan*, 62.

[71] Indra, *Swapnadosh Vigyan*, 64.

[72] For discussion on reproduction, brahmacharya, and the notion of eugenics, see Veronika Fuechtner, Douglas E. Haynes, and Ryan M. Jones (ed.), *A Global History of Sexual Science, 1880–1960* (California: University of California Press, 2018). For details on same sex love, see Ruth Vanita and Saleem Kidwai (eds), *Same Sex Love in India* (Palgrave, New York, 2000).

[73] For details, see Judith E. Walsh, *Domesticity in Colonial India: What Women Learned When Men Gave Them Advice* (New York: Rowman and Littlefield Publishers, 2004); Judith E. Walsh, *How to Be the Goddess of Your Home: An Anthology of Bengali Domestic Manuals* (New Delhi: Yoda Press, 2005); Ann Laura Stoler, 'Making Empire Respectable: The Politics of Race and Sexual Morality in 20th-Century Colonial Cultures', *American Ethnologist*, vol. 16, no. 4 (1989): 634–60; Tanika Sarkar, *Hindu Wife, Hindu Nation*

the complex hegemony of nationalist and rationalist thoughts that governed concerns of well-being, progress, and future of the nation state. Medicine, therefore, cannot be situated outside the domains of social and cultural histories of the period. The health of the Hindu nation came to be irreplaceably linked to men's ability to control their desires, whereas women's reproductive abilities were concurrent with the future of the nation. National politics and sexual health were inextricably tied to each other. Men and semen were regarded to be superior; their desires and lust became part of the national debate. Women, on the other hand, were desexualized. While there was unabated debates on men, masturbation, and bodily predilections, the issue of female masturbation was almost never discussed. Female sexual health and hygiene were at the centre stage because of their reproductive capabilities. Nonetheless, there are few instances wherein female desire came under scrutiny. Hysteria or *yoshapasmar* was one such disease and it was believed to occur in women who had pleasure-seeking tendencies.

Hysteria as a disease is regarded to be protean in its content and form. Historians working on the disease are often baffled by its rise and fall. It acquired enormous attention by the mad-doctors, alienists, and later psychiatrists till the beginning of the twentieth century. Jean Charcot and his famous disciple Sigmund Freud made their careers with the theatrics of hysterics. By the late 1930s, the diagnosis of hysteria had faded from the alleged taxonomies of madness. In the context of India, the disease witnessed its emergence only in the first few decades of the twentieth century. This delay can be understood due to the postponement of the transfer of knowledge of health and disease and its acceptance and eventual dissemination in the colonies. Hysteria was called yoshapasmar in Sanskrit and Hindi. It was named such because the symptoms of hysteria were regarded to be similar to epileptic fits or *apasmar*.

There exist few references on hysteria in Hindi medical literature. One such significant essay is 'Hysteria ya Yoshapasmar' (hysteria or yoshapasmar) published in the journal *Aarogya-Vigyan* in 1933, which

Community: Religion and Cultural Nationalism (Delhi: Permanent Black, 2001); Sumit Sarkar, 'The "Women's Question" in Nineteenth Century Bengal', in Women and Culture, edited by Kumkum Sangari and Sudesh Vaid (Bombay: Research Centre for Women's Studies, 1994), 103–12, among others.

was written by Indiradevi.[74] She claimed herself to be a learned vaidya. She argues:

> Hysteria does not share similar symptoms with any of the mentioned and elaborately described diseases within the nomenclature of the Ancient ayurvedic texts such as Charak, Sushrut, etc. That is why while some of the medical men consider it as madness, others regard it as a form of anxiety or epilepsy. But because this is specific to women, it cannot be associated with these general mental diseases.[75]

It is, therefore, clear that the emergence of hysteria as a disease in Hindi medical literature was a result of the intermeshing of Western and indigenous ideas. While Indiradevi referred to hysteria as yoshapasmar, the general medical textbooks used the English term 'hysteria' itself. The English term 'hysteria' in the north Indian context referred to a generalized concept of female insanity. The association, although generalized, also had a specific meaning in the period under study.

Indiradevi pointed out that 'although women by mind, body and nature are selfless, women who have pleasure seeking (*rajasik*) tendencies are prone to this disease. This is generally caused due to problems related to womb and mental illness. Sometimes anxiety or weakness of brain can also be the cause of this disease'.[76] According to the Ayurvedic concept, manas or mind has three basic qualities. These were based on the idea that food had the capacity to alter human character. These are *satwik*, rajasik, and *tamsik*. Satwik or *satwa* refers to self-control and knowledge which is because of consumption of pure food. Rajasik refers to a self-loving, pleasure-seeking, and authoritarian person. A tamsik person is dull and inactive.[77] The selflessness of women was a trope based on which the story of Indian motherhood was usually woven. Women, in other words, were regarded as less sexual than men. This idea gave the nationalistic discourse an upper hand to control and manage

---

[74] Indiradevi, *Hysteria ya Yoshapasmar, Aarogya Vigyan*, part 2, no. 5 (February 1933).

[75] Indiradevi, *Hysteria ya Yoshapasmar*, 417.

[76] Indiradevi, *Hysteria ya Yoshapasmar*, 418.

[77] Dinesh Bhugra, 'Psychiatry in Ancient Indian Texts: A Review', *History of Psychiatry*, vol. 3 (1992): 170.

women's sexuality. The desire-less woman was easy to be tamed and managed by marriage and motherhood as soon as she reached puberty. Therefore, any rajasik tendencies in women were considered unnatural making them prone to hysteria. The marriageable age of women was considered to be a matter of extreme importance and any interference from the colonial Fovernment agitated Indian nationalists because they regarded the issue to be sacred to their community, religion, and nation. The age of consent debates have been discussed in detail by historians working on gender in colonial India.[78]

The womb as a cause of female insanity has been debated since ancient times. Elaine Showalter argues that 'for centuries, hysteria had been the quintessential female malady, the very name of which derived from the Greek hysteron, or womb'.[79] The idea of the 'wandering womb' linked to women's insanity was novel in the Indian context. Indiradevi also remarked that 'if the early symptoms of "yoshopasmar" are visible in an adult girl then the intelligent Vaidya should advice her parents to marry her as early as possible. Patients start showing signs of recovery soon after the marriage with basic treatment'.[80] Marriage as an ubiquitous cure for madness continued to be offered by ojhas, shamans, and vaidyas. This notion is again gendered and women are often advised to marry if they show symptoms of insanity. Sudhir Kakar, while discussing the pir of Pattershah Dargah, describes the case of a woman suffering from mental health issues, which was narrated by the baba to him:

'There was another young girl,' Baba continued, 'very beautiful and innocent-looking, who used to come to me with her father. In her dreams too a man came and incited her to the bad act. The girl did not agree to

---

[78] For a detailed discussion on the age of consent, see Dagmar Engels, 'The Age of Consent Act of 1891: Colonial Ideology in Bengal', *South Asia Research*, vol. 3, no. 2 (1983): 107–31; Tanika Sarkar, 'Rhetoric against Age of Consent: Resisting Colonial Reason and Death of a Child-Wife', *Economic and Political Weekly*, vol. 28, no. 36 (1993): 1869–78; Tanika Sarkar, 'A Prehistory of Rights: The Age of Consent Debate in Colonial Bengal', *Feminist Studies*, vol. 26, no. 3 (2000): 601–22, among others.

[79] Showalter, *The Female Malady*, 129.

[80] Indiradevi, *Hysteria ya Yoshapasmar*, 419.

the man's proposition, but she could not fall asleep at night for the fear that the bad act might be done to her unawares while she slept. I gave her "holy water" and there was an improvement in her condition. But after a few days some other man started appearing in her dreams and making the same demand. Night after night, the girl lay awake ... Now I know why she cannot sleep and falls ill every day. All these demons waiting to enter her house one after another! I told her father to marry her off immediately. After marriage when she is with a man, the demons will leave her and find someone else. The father followed my advice and now the girl is perfectly alright.'[81]

The baba's solution to marry the girl off remains a common practice. The idea is widespread due to several reasons. First, it was commonly believed from ancient times that women's unsatisfied sexual appetites could drive them mad. A woman's inability to control herself is due to the frail nature of her body. Channelling her body and sexuality towards a man could cure her physical and mental ailments. Second, any bizarre behaviour on the part of women which included her conscious and unconscious desires to seek sexual pleasure shook the morality of Indian society in which women (and often men) were not expected to express their need for sexual gratification. The solution, therefore, of the problem was to marry the girl off as soon as possible.

Indiradevi asserted that 'unmarried girls, child widows and barren women are more prone to yoshapasmar. This disease is usually not found in women who have children and are faithful to their husband. This is why this disease is considered to be a sort of insanity.'[82] Moral conditioning of the men and women became the utmost primary duty of the indigenous medical practitioners. Health, body, and above all sexuality, were intimately tied to the nation-building project. Scholars working on modern Ayurveda have reiterated that during the colonial period an urgent need for the glorification of the past was felt to rescue, resuscitate, and revitalize the present with the glory of the past. Gupta remarks that by the early twentieth century most vaidyas in the colonial United Provinces chose Hindi as their primary language of

---

[81] Sudhir Kakar, *Shamans, Mystics, and Doctors: A Psychological Inquiry into India and Its Healing Traditions* (Delhi: Oxford University Press, 1992), 21.

[82] Indiradevi, *Hysteria ya Yoshapasmar*, 418.

dialogue.[83] The ancient past was invoked as the great age of Ayurveda while the present *kaliyuga* was blamed for its declining status.[84] Gupta has interestingly discussed the case of Yashoda Devi who she called herself a 'moral sexologist'.[85] Yashoda Devi's expertise was to cure women's sexual and reproductive ailments. Gupta has pointed out that 'sexuality engaged her constant attention, and was seen by her in scientific, medical and moralistic terms. Her books constantly talked of her clients' sexual lives. *Dampatya Prem* (1933) was specifically devoted to it. She stressed that sexual science and passionate intercourse was an intrinsic part of ayurveda'.[86]

Yashoda Devi was unique as she acknowledged the significance of women's desires. Nonetheless, vaidyas saw women (more often than men) as reproductive devices whose desire for intimacy had to be sublimated into the accepted models of motherhood. Indiradevi's ideas on women's faithfulness is one of those necessary claims which was not exclusively to be found in her writings. Gupta remarked, 'There was a reordering of the ideas of household and conjugality alongside images of an idealized wife imbued with reformist endeavour, and sexual disciplining and control over the woman's body and hersocial movements.'[87] Hysteria as a disease in the nineteenth century could be regarded as an innovative label used in Western countries and later in India to ascribe and pathologize women who transgressed societal boundaries. Roy Porter while discussing hysteria noted, 'There were intense pressures towards inculcating self-control, self-discipline and outward conformity (bourgeois respectability). Personal responsibility, probity and piety were, furthermore, internalized through strict moral training, imparted via hallowed socialization agencies like family, neighbourhood, school

---

[83]   Charu Gupta, 'Procreation and Pleasure: Writings of a Woman Ayurvedic Practitioner in Colonial North India', *Studies in History*, vol. 21, no. 1 (2005): 21

[84]   Gupta, 'Procreation and Pleasure': 21.

[85]   Gupta, 'Procreation and Pleasure': 20. For more information on *kaliyuga*, see Sumit Sarkar, '"Kaliyuga", "Chakri" and "Bhakti": Ramakrishna and His Times', *Economic and Political Weekly*, vol. 27, no. 29 (18 July 1992): 1543–59 and 1561–6.

[86]   Gupta, 'Procreation and Pleasure': 32.

[87]   Gupta, 'Procreation and Pleasure': 29.

and chapel.'[88] While in India these class-based rules were amiss to some extent, diseases often were carriers of ideas that earlier had not found ground in Indian scenario. The transference of these diseases brought formally fashioned ideas around them. In the West, hysteria had an entrenched relationship with gender and class. Its reconfiguration in India led to the reformulation of some of these ideas while others were transferred with its inane biases.

Indiradevi argued,

> Those young women, who are delicate, fashionable, refrain from physical activities, habitual of reading romantic novels, adulteress, and also those who failed to achieve the object of their affection or who are by their bodily constitution anxious are prone to this disease. Besides, overindulgence in food and sexual pleasures, and problems related to menstruation, constipation, indigestion, etc. also cause this disease.[89]

Pleasure, sexual or derived from any other source, became a target of those who claimed to cure hysteria. In other words, what came under attack was the upper-middle-class lifestyle as it supposedly degenerated women's moral, mental, and physical constitution leaving them mad. The discussion has similar connotations, which one has already witnessed, in case of men who go astray, masturbate, and lose their mental balance by deriving pleasure from activities which were regarded as amoral by the indigenous vaidyas of the period. Hysteria has been regarded as a class-based disease in the Western context as well. The illness found its niche among the upper-class or upper-middle-class women who were so prone to pleasure. They lost moral standings and fell to the level of prostitutes. Andrew Scull pointed out that 'paragons of moral obliquity, most hysterical women were thus blameworthy, not sick. They were actresses, not real invalids, and yet they clung to their symptoms with a fierceness and persistence that defied and defeated most medical men's efforts to cure them.'[90]

---

[88] Roy Porter, 'The Body and the Mind, the Doctor and the Patient: Negotiating Hysteria', in *Hysteria Beyond Freud*, edited by Sander L. Gilman, Helen King, et al. (Berkley: University of California Press, 2003), 229.

[89] Indiradevi, *Hysteria ya Yoshapasmar*, 418.

[90] Andrew Scull, *Hysteria: The Biography* (Oxford: Oxford University Press, 2009), 69.

Moral depravity was a sin against the Hindu nation. Medical discourses were full of directions to achieve righteous living fused with codes to assist the building of health, vitality, and nation building. Pleasures sought from food or sex were not merely immoral but completely unacceptable in times of nationalist struggle.[91] Therefore, diseases such as hysteria (attacking women who were prone to pleasure) and masturbation (attacking men who lacked self-control) were troubles that reflected class, community, and national predicaments. Kavita Sivaramakrishnan's work on Ayurveda in colonial Punjab highlights that 'colonial medicine, therefore, was shaped by the specific exigencies of Indian environment and culture.'[92] This is not to deny that ancient Indian texts did not have misogynist leanings.[93] Shalini Shah has looked at the representation of female sexuality in the Ayurvedic discourses of the early medieval period. She remarks that 'given the social reality, women's body both in health and pleasure, had no autonomy of expression but was depended on male guardian or physician for its manifestation.'[94] She further pointed out that 'when these ayurvedic treatise deals with women's pathology, it is with disease pertaining to the uterus.'[95] Nevertheless, the advent of

---

[91] For details, see Saadat Hasan Manto's story 'Swaraj ke liye' in which he questions the idea of sexual restrain and patriotism (Saadat Hasan Manto, 'For Freedom's Sake', in *Black Margins*, edited by Muhammad Umar Memon, translated into English by M. Asaduddin (Oxford University Press, 2001), 105–34.

[92] Kavita Sivramakrishnan, 'Constructing Boundaries, Contesting Identities: The Politics of Ayurved in Punjab (1930–1940)', *Studies in History*, vol. 22, no. 2 (2006): 254.

[93] For details, see Kumkum Roy, *The Power of Gender and the Gender of Power: Explorations in Early Indian History* (Oxford University Press, New Delhi, 2010); Rahul Peter Das, *The Origin of the Life of a Human Being: Conception and the Female According to Ancient Medical and Sexological Literature* (Delhi: Motilal Banarsidass Publishers Private Limited, 2003); Daud Ali, 'Aristocratic Body Techniques in Early Medieval India', in *Rethinking a Millennium*, edited by Rajat Dutta (Delhi: Aakar Books, 2008), 25–56.

[94] Shalini Shah, 'Representation of Female Sexuality in the Ayurvedic Discourse of the Early Medieval Period', *Studies in History*, vol. 22, no. 1 (2006): 48.

[95] Shah, 'Representation of Female Sexuality': 48.

colonialism followed by aggressive nationalism saw the entrenchment of patriarchal authority in a modern way.

These ideas had interesting afterlives and continued to resurface in the following decades. A published text from the 1960s entitled *Dehati Chikitsak* or local healer, published by Hamdard reiterated,

> The disease [hysteria] is usually found among urban, delicate and rich women but sometimes it also occurs in women from rural areas. Generally this occurs in women who refrain from doing physical work, lead a life of pleasures and those who have interest in reading love stories. Sometimes, digestion problem, constipation, sorrow, anger and fear can also lead to the fits of Hysteria.[96]

The text further describes,

> the fits of hysteria can stay from few minutes to some hours and this usually occurs after the menstruation. Patient usually experiences headache before the fit. Eyes start to get watery and the body suffers from weakness. After sometime, a ball of air starts to rise from stomach and gets struck in the throat. Then the patient tries to swallow and clear the throat but she fails and starts to feel breathless. She tries to burp but her heartbeats increase and suffer from frequent urination.[97]

Indiradevi's description lacked the details of symptoms which were delineated in detail in *Dehati Chikitsak*.

This description echoed the symptomology given by Galen. Scull notes,

> Both Soranus and Galen, by contrast, disputed the notion that the womb could wander, though they accepted that it was the organ from which hysterical symptoms derived. These manifestations of the disease could take a multitude of forms: extreme emotionality; but also a variety of physical disturbances, ranging from simple dizziness, through paralyses, and respiratory distress. Then there was the commonly reported sensation of a ball in the throat, constricting breathing and creating a sense of suffocation, the so-called *globus hystericus*. There was thus a venerable

---

[96] *Dehati Chikitsak*, part 2 (Hamdard Publication, n.d.).
[97] *Dehati Chikitsak*, part 2, 201.

tradition within Western medicine that linked hysteria to gender—and perhaps even to sexuality, for Galen held that sexual deprivation could cause the disorder, and advocated intercourse for the married, and marriage for the single, as a frequently valuable therapeutic tactic.[98]

Following the lead of great masters, *Dehati Chikitsak* also cautioned that 'girls who have not been married till late and those who have excessive sexual desires are prone to this disease' (see Figure 5.3).[99] It further mentioned that 'the patient starts to shout and cry, and then suddenly burst into laughter and becomes unconscious [*sic*]'.[100]

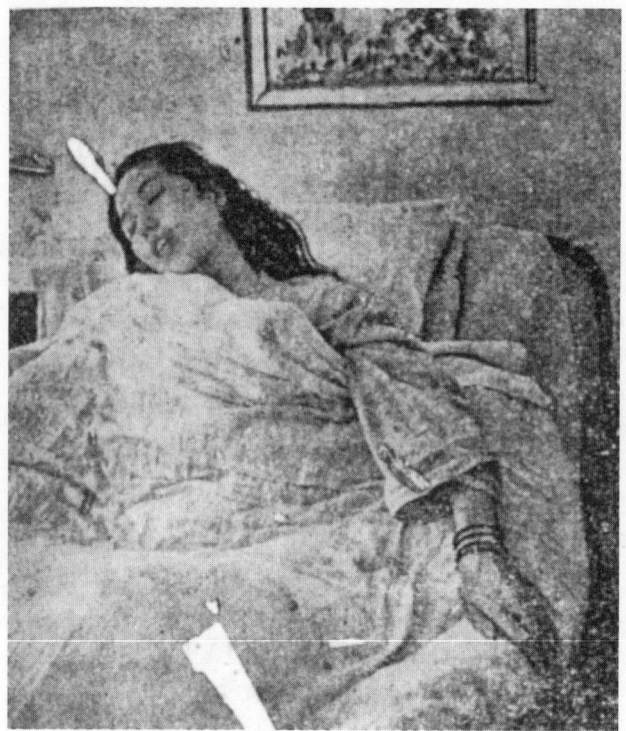

Figure 5.3   Girl suffering from hysteria; image from *Dehati Chikitsak*
Source: Hindi Nagari Pracharani Sabha, Collection.

[98] Scull, *Hysteria: The Biography*, 16.
[99] *Dehati Chikitsak*, part 2, 200–1.
[100] *Dehati Chikitsak*, part 2, 202.

While discussing printed discourses and circulation of ideas on reproduction in early modern Europe, Mary E. Fissell points out, 'The advent of print had unexpected consequences for ideas about women's bodies.'[101] She also argues that 'the transmission of that knowledge outwards is, in this model, always imperfect and corrupting'.[102] The beginning of the twentieth century also saw an upsurge in Hindi print media with far-reaching consequences. Hindi books, pamphlets, and advertisements were circulated among the higher and the lower castes and classes. Hindi medical books for everyday cures were widely available at the time. These ideas and practices became a formidable arsenal during the nationalist struggle. What is interesting to note is that some of these ideas such as hysteria were products of the exchange between indigenous and Western medicine. Exchange as a process was not simply implementation of Western medicine, rather it was complicated involving vernacularization and dissemination, which included contestation and segregation of ideas that reflected the needs of the time. Mukharji asserts that vernacularization as a process was not simply 'the rendering of something into a "vernacular" language. Rather it is the process of creatively adapting a knowledge and its attendant practices to fit a new historical context'.[103]

Hysteria was regarded to be a chameleon-like disease which had characteristics that defied easy diagnosis, prognosis, and cure. Eminent physicians attempted to treat it with new technological inventions which left an indelible mark on the history of womanhood. These included intrusive, painful, and penalizing surgeries which attempted to erase any sort of pleasure from sex, leaving their bodies disabled. Clitoridectomy, ovariotomy, and finally electric vibrators were all used to treat women suffering from hysteria. It is difficult to ascertain the extent to which hysteria was diagnosed by the hakims, vaidyas, or other healers. Neither was hysteria a popular diagnosis in the asylum records. The reason

---

[101] Mary E. Fissell, *Vernacular Bodies: The Politics of Reproduction in Early Modern England* (Oxford: Oxford University Press, 2004), 3

[102] Fissell, *Vernacular Bodies*, 6.

[103] Projit B. Mukharji, 'Vernacularizing the Body: Informational Egalitarianism, Hindu Divine Design and Race in Physiology School Books, Bengal 1859–1877', *Bulletin of the History of Medicine*, vol. 91, no. 3 (2017): 556.

behind it could be that it was after all an illness of civilized, urban, and sophisticated women. Asylums, as argued, were houses of poor and dangerous for the most part of the colonial period. The notion of hysteria, therefore, thrived more outside the walled lives of asylums. Indrani Sen notes that 'discursive colonial writings do seem to indicate that mental health problems among white women were quite high. Problems such as nervous breakdown, depression, hysteria and homesickness were widely prevalent and one comes across repeated references to these conditions. These problems are said to have been frequently found among middle-class European women.'[104]

The disease and the label had long and interesting afterlives. Whether it is hysteria or masturbation, their delayed dissemination resulted in their myth-like re-emergence in the psychiatric repertory. It was not the indigenous healers who often used these categories in everyday practice; well-qualified psychiatrists continue to write, publish, and diagnose patients with these so-called ailments. Sarah Pinto remarks in her medical anthropological work on psychiatry in contemporary times that 'in the large government clinic many young women, married and unmarried were diagnosed with dissociative disorder, an ailment clinicians usually referred as "hysteria." These women were treated with pharmaceuticals and subjected to disciplinary techniques involving spouses, parents and in-laws, who were instructed not to respond to their demands. Few such diagnoses were made in private clinic.'[105] Delayed arrival of these categories, along with their corrupted scientific reimaging because of their nationalistic acquisitions, had intrinsic disciplinary measures redefining gender roles wherein transgressions were handed down with subterfuge labels leading to long-term consequences.

***

Emergence of the 'mind sciences' in vernacular Hindi literature was a variegated phenomenon. While Western ideas on madness impacted

[104] Indrani Sen, 'The Memsahib's "Madness": The European Woman's Mental Health in Late Nineteenth Century India', *Social Scientist*, vol. 33, nos 5–6 (May–June 2005): 33.

[105] Sarah Pinto, *Daughters of Parvati: Women and Madness in Contemporary India* (Philadelphia: University of Pennsylvania Press, 2014), 22.

the ways in which insanity was understood in late nineteenth- and early twentieth-century colonial India, a complicated process of segregation and filtration was involved. Certain categories were fused with ancient wisdom and new taxonomies of madness emerged. The meanings were altered and cures offered intended self-disciplining and gendered aligning to alter society. This was not very different from the Western context. Historians working on madness have often pointed towards the inherent relationship between the emergence of psychiatric knowledge and the exerted social control. Hindi sources directly dealing with insanity are very sparse. There is an urgent need to diversify our sources in order to further examine how 'the power of mind' emerged as a potent category to cure what nationalists regarded as a phase of national 'impotency'. After all, 'pathologization of mind' occurred in a very different way. Insanity was regarded more as a 'collective pathology' than an 'individual sickness' in the colonial period. The body as a metaphor for the nation has been discussed in detail by numerous historical works. The mind and its sickness have received little attention so far. The yogic feats, attempts to find a panacea that could cure all illnesses, and belief in a 'supreme Aryan race' were pathologies that need to be interrogated from the point of view of both mind and body in order to understand what Fanon called the 'violence of colonialism'.

Epilogue

The Pakistani soldiers caught hold of him and tried to push towards the other side, but he refused to move, 'Toba Tek Singh is here!' And then he raised his voice, 'Opar di gurgur di annexe di bay dhiana di mung di daal of Toba Tek Singh and Pakistan.' ... Just before sunrise, a sky rending cry emerged from the gullet of Bishen Singh, who till then had stood still and unmoving. Several officials came running to the spot and found that the man who had stood on his leg, day and night for fifteen years, was lying on his face. Over there, behind the barbed wires, was Hindustan. Over here, behind identical wires lay Pakistan. In between, on a bit of land that had no name, lay Toba Tek Singh.[1]

In Saadat Hussain Manto's short story 'Toba Tek Singh', when news of the exchange of inmates of the lunatic asylums between the newly created nations Hindustan and Pakistan reached the

[1] Saadat Hasan Manto, 'Toba Tek Singh', in *Black Margins*, edited by Muhammad Umar Memon, translated by English by M. Asaduddin (Katha: Oxford University Press, 2001), 220.

hospital, it led to quite a commotion. It had been decided that the Sikh and the Hindu inmates would be sent from Pakistan to India and the Muslim inmates of the asylums in India would be transported to Pakistan. The bewildered patients started discussing where would be the respective locations of Pakistan and Hindustan. This was a question that the governments themselves had not been able to settle easily. A patient named Bishen Singh tries to resolve the mystery of Hindustan/ Pakistan but fails. He was interested in his land, a place called Toba Tek Singh. When Bishen Singh failed to comprehend the location of Toba Tek Singh as he had no conception of a communal geographical divide, he refused to move and died between the two countries. The larger question that the story poses is whether the real lunatics are within or outside the asylums.

The short stories of Saadat Hasan Manto (1912–1955) are the most powerful literary representations of the horrors of the Partition violence. The extract in the epigraph is from his famous story 'Toba Tek Singh', written from the perspective of eponymous inmate of the Lahore Mental Hospital, and widely regarded as one of the most moving accounts of the Partition ever written. Manto's provocative story was also a reflection of reality in a literal sense since an exchange of lunatics actually took place after the Partition. The Annual Report of the Punjab Mental Hospital, Amritsar, for the Year 1950 stated:

> Four hundred, and Fifty non-Muslim mental patients were received from Lahore out of which 282 Punjabi patients were accommodated in the Amritsar Mental Hospital, the remaining having been sent to the Inter-Provincial Mental Hospital, Ranchi. As against this 233 Muslim patients were evacuated in the opposite direction to Lahore. That against an esti-mated non-Muslim population of six to seven hundred of the Mental Hospital, Lahore at the time of partition only 317 patients were actu-ally exchanged at the time of transfer, is a tragic fact which sadly betrays the treatment meted out to those unfortunate victims who could not be retrieved earlier from the Lahore Hospital.[2]

Around 300 to 400 patients died in a period of three years, while many more died on the way from Lahore to Amritsar. There exists no mention,

---

[2] The Annual Report on the Working of Punjab Mental Hospital Amritsar for the year 1950, NAI.

forget any sort of commemoration, of the sufferings of mourning lunatics except for this brief description of these 'unfortunate' victims. This was because they were insane, and being insane meant being 'lesser humans' who did not deserve or need any attention whatsoever. Manto's story is one about the madness of Partition and the lunatics who perpetrated its attended violence. Bishen Singh and the other 'lunatics' were saner than the governments of Britain, India, and Pakistan. The madness of the violence of the Partition was a result of the madness of colonialism.

The Lahore asylum was one of the largest in north India. It has been central to this book due to its historical significance and tryst with Partition (see Figure E.1). Nonetheless, for a long time I was not able to visit Pakistan due to animosity between the country and India. The invitation to present my paper at the International Conference for Historians of Asia in Islamabad (5–9 December 2016) provided me with the wonderful opportunity to visit Lahore for research. A kind Pakistani embassy official's respect for historical scholarship helped open the

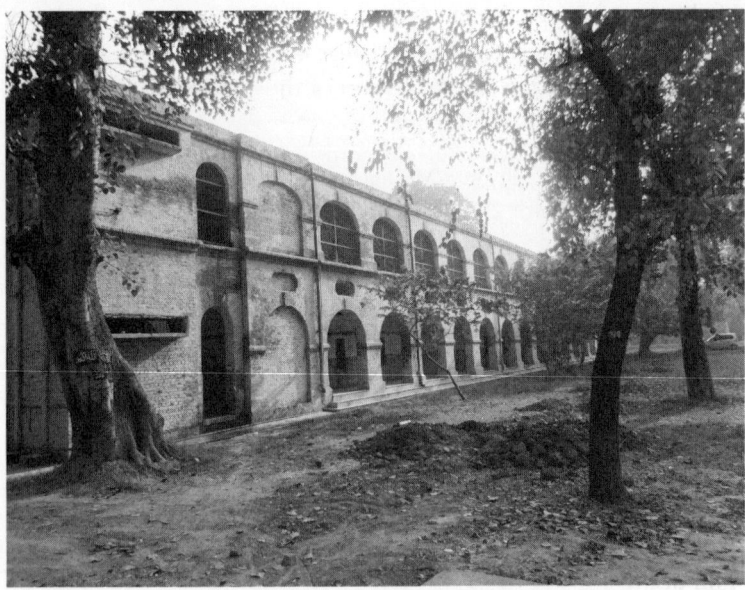

Figure E.1   The Lahore Mental Hospital, photographed in 2016
Source: Author.

doors of the Lahore Mental Asylum to this harmless academic. There exists no 'research' or 'academic' visa for citizens to travel between the two countries. All those who work on Punjab's history end up only looking at the material on either side of the border. The concept of facilitating 'scholars across borders' has not yet seeped into the psyches of the respective belligerent governments. The result is that all those who work on the many myriad subjects that unite Indians and Pakistanis—for example, the history of the Indus Valley civilization or undivided Punjab—rarely get a chance to conduct fieldwork in either nation.

My unconscious desire to cross the border was shaped by longings of my great-grandparents and grandparents who continue to still live their lives in the time capsule of that moment when their homeland became an 'enemy' nation. My rationale was formed, however, with childhood stories alongside the ontological/historical/rational 'self' of a trained modern Indian historian. Amid increasing tensions between India and Pakistan, I got the rarest of opportunities to visit the other side of the border. I was aware that Manto, who wrote about the Lahore asylum was also hospitalized there several times. Conscious of this fact, I spent hours carefully screening through the material, when suddenly I came across Manto's name and address. I was over the moon! For a historian researching the history of madness in South Asia this was nothing short of discovering the Kohinoor diamond after a long and arduous treasure hunt.

The record is incomplete as it only had a sentence mentioning his name, his father's name and address along with a line stating that his admission was 'voluntary' or razakar. A plausible reason for the incomplete nature of the record could be to save Manto from the disgrace of being an alcoholic or 'insane'. Further, the tradition of proper record-keeping had also declined soon after the British left. This phenomenon again is remarkably similar across South Asian borders. Finding Manto's name made my visit to Pakistan simultaneously more memorable and poignant. Manto epitomized the tragedy of the Partition. His decision to migrate was taken due to pressure from his family members who had moved to Pakistan. Increasing communal tensions in India had left him disheartened. He left for Pakistan in the hope of receiving proper recognition. Far from being acknowledged, after his move, Manto failed to even manage a job. His financial struggle, increasing court cases, and disillusionment with Pakistan drove him towards alcoholism. He died broken and disillusioned on 12 January 1955. Manto died a decade before the first India–Pakistan war in 1965 and also before jingoism became the lingua franca between these two nations.

This book has probed the madness of colonialism that attempted organization and management of human insanity. This madness ended with the mayhem of the Partition. The confinement of lunacy to the lunatic asylums reflected benevolence and philanthropy of the colonial state but what could not be confined was the violence of colonialism. The asylums emerged as locations where the mad and the 'debauched' (ganja, charas, and opium smokers along with the 'others' who were seen as deviant, such as faqirs) were locked up. There was a constant rhetoric of reform which never became a reality. The continued use of jails points towards the limits of colonial psychiatry. The Report of the Indian Hemp Drugs Commission led to the reorganization of the lunatic asylums. Several smaller lunatic asylums were merged with the larger ones. Such mammoth asylums, in the absence of modern facilities, soon became unmanageable. The study of psychiatry never emerged as a specialized discipline. Few specialists (European or Indian) though were sent to England, Europe, and America for training in the discipline. The architecture of colonial asylums shows that these institutions were built more or less as 'glorified prisons'. The diagnosis and categories reveal the fuzziness of colonial psychiatry. Diagnosis depended on classifying the patients as either 'dangerous' or 'curable'. Categories were often simplistic and medically irrelevant. A closer look at the low status of the Indian staff indicates that there was not much difference between them and patients within the asylum hierarchy. The two worked in close coopera-tion at times while at other times were antagonistic to each other. The focus on the banal lives of inmates has demonstrated the fact that the patients often had to work hard in order to survive within these institu-tions. 'Hard working' and 'well behaved' lunatics were rewarded through allowance of additional food and money. The lives of patients and those of the lower-level Indian staff became bearable because of the diverse recreation provided in the asylum.

The study of case histories reflected that the patients belonging to dif-ferent strata of society were lodged in these institutions. The prevalent notions about gender, caste, and class often coloured the diagnosis and treatment of the patients. We have also seen that by the early twentieth century, the Indian middle class had internalized Western notions of 'sanity' and 'insanity'. The mental hospitals catered to the needs of this burgeoning middle class by offering them separate rooms. The category of paid patients emerges as an important one in the hospital records. Families often played an important role in the incarceration of their 'deviant' relatives.

In the course of this research I have analysed various psychiatric ideas and their prevalence and popularity at different times, individual cases or case histories, the politics of psychiatric practices, quotidian histories of the asylums, and the lunacy laws. In other words, at the macro level, a close look at legislation and inquiries has helped in unravelling the processes involved in the homogenization, medicalization, and professionalization of psychiatric infrastructure. At the micro level, it has focused on the lives of the patients. It has looked at everyday histories of the asylums. Routine activities such as 'employment and amusement', 'diet and medicine', and 'reform and reward', among others, were constitutive of the asylum's regime.

The study of case histories enhanced understandings of doctor–patient interactions, and aided in bringing out the coercive as well as the therapeutic aspects of 'colonial' psychiatry. It has been argued that over the period of a century psychiatry came to provide the political, social, educational, and legal framework for locating the 'normal' and the civilized who had a firm faith in British modernity, medicine, and science. At the same time the study reveals that the psychiatric infrastructure was conspicuously limited and underdeveloped even on the eve of Independence and that postcolonial India had to grapple with the legacy of these inadequacies. The emergence of professionalized psychiatry created a milieu where a plethora of healing practices and beliefs were regarded as primitive and superstitious charlatanism. More recently, psychiatrists and psychologists have come to accept the significance of healing cultures to the local members of communities who had little or no access to Western medical treatment. It has been proven that faith, socio-religious practices, and healing are often essential for recovery and well-being of those suffering from mental illness. On the other hand, many psychiatric practices including that of lobotomy and ECT have become redundant.

This book has attempted to bring together rather disjointed world views of 'scientific' and religious, institutionalized and non-institutionalized, and colonial and nationalistic ideas on curing madness. The book, however, is limited to institutional record and select Hindi medical literature on mental illness. Future projects will benefit from the incorporation of Urdu and Punjabi medical literature on the subject.

Appendices

Appendix 1

Name- Sadhu Jalender Nath	**Age-** 35 years
Caste- Hindu Faqir	**Occupation-** Beggar
Received from- Orai	**Date of Admission-** 21.6.07
Mental Disease- Dementia	**Cause-**
Result of Treatment- Died on 29.12.52 at 1.30. A.M	
Health on Admission- Fair	**Weight-** 114
Health on Discharge-	**Weight-**
Residence-	**Vaccination-**

[The case notes of the patient are only available from 7.9.46]

Date	Notes on the Cases
7.9.46	123 lbs, dull, blind, no work
16.10.46	125 lbs, do, do, do
6.11.46	123 lbs, do, do, do
2.12.46	121 lbs, hospital
4.1.47	120 lbs, do
11.3.47	126 lbs, infirm, old
10.4.47	121 lbs, no work, infirm
8.5. 47	128 lbs, no work, infirm
5.6. 47	130 lbs
7.7.47	132 lbs
5.8.47	133 lbs
9.9.47	132 lbs, he is infirm, gang. He is blind in both eyes. There is no melancholy
4.10.47	135 lbs, old infirm, no work
5.11.47	132 lbs, do
2.12.47	130 lbs, does not see properly, do
7.1.48	129 lbs, chronic dementia, no work, can't see
16.2.48	128 lbs, old infirm, dementia, no work
3.3.48	124 lbs, old infirm, dementia, no work
6.4.48	124 lbs, old infirm, chronic dementia, no work
17.5.48	126 lbs, chronic dementia, no work
10.6.48	126 lbs, old and infirm
7.7.48	128 lbs, old infirm, cannot see, cataract, no work
16.8.48	129 lbs, old and infirm, cataract, no work
6.9.48	134 lbs, old and infirm, cataract, no work
8.10.48	130 lbs, chronic dementia, unable to work, anxiety of old age
6.11.48	131 lbs, [illegible] no change
6.12.48	135 lbs, old and infirm, cannot see [illegible]
5.1.49	136 lbs, old infirm, no work
10.2.49	137 lbs, do, do
7.3.49	138 lbs, do, do
7.4.49	137 lbs, do, do
9.6.49	136 lbs
13.7.49	137 lbs

Date	Notes on the Cases
8.8.49	136 lbs
8.9.49	134 lbs
10.10.49	130 lbs
9.11.49	137 lbs
12.12.49	134 lbs
18.1.50	134 lbs
14.2.50	136 lbs
26.3.50	134 lbs
28. 3.50	137 lbs
20.6. 50	132 lbs
14.7.50	128 lbs
12.8.50	126 lbs
11.9.50	123 lbs
19.10.50	124 lbs
15.11.50	123 lbs
20.12.50	131 lbs
23.1.51	118 lbs
20.2.51	120 lbs
20.3.51	120 lbs
24.4.51	114 lbs
25.5.51	120 lbs
24.6.51	119 lbs
28.7.51	120 lbs
30.8.51	120 lbs
30.9.51	121 lbs, he has got cataract in his both eyes. He is very old now
2. 11.51	122 lbs
18.11.51	123 lbs
24.1.52	123 lbs, quiet
22.2.52	120 lbs, quiet
6.3.52	114 lbs, fever, admitted infirmary, very senile
22.4.52	118 lbs, [illegible] feeble heart
5.5.52	106 lbs, losing weight
10.6.52	100 lbs, losing weight

Date	Notes on the Cases
23.7.52	98 lbs, he is continuing losing weight. He often gets some rise in temp daily in evening. He is markedly anaemic
24.7.52	98 lbs
26.7.52	[The case notes between 26.7.52 to 29.12.52 are missing]

Expired on 29.12.52

Appendix 2

Name- Rashid s/o Faizal Hakim Khan	**Age-** 47
Caste- Mohamedan	**Occupation-** Vagrant
Received from- Transferred from M. H. Benares	**Date of Admission-** 5.12.42
Mental Disease- Dementia	**Cause-**
Result of Treatment-	**Health on Admission-** Fair
Weight- 87 lbs	**Health on Discharge-**
Weight-	**Residence-** Sadr bazaar homeless. ['Not known' was struck off and replaced with 'Sadr Bazaar homeless' in the original case register]

Marks of Identification- Shallow   **Vaccination-**
scar on inner the middle [illegible]
of left forearm. A scar on the left
leg below the knee

Copy of Medical Certificate- He after facing his head upwards abuses the deputy superintendent, says that it has snatched his wife though he was never married, does no work, whatsoever, remains roaming and murmuring in his cell all the day.

Signed
V.S. Gupta
Captain
B.Sc. MBBS
Superintendent. District Jail, Meerut

Date	Notes on the Cases

Tongue, Clean & moist
Heart, no murmur heard
Lungs, Clean B.S. Vericulum
Lungs and Spleen, not palpable

[Dates of the case notes are missing]

88 lbs, quiet, no work
90 lbs, do, do
90 lbs, do, do
93 lbs, do, do
92 lbs, dull, no work
94 lbs, dull, no work
96 lbs, quiet, do
97 lbs, do, do
88 lbs, ill, no work, weak
86 lbs, ill nourished, weak lungs, head and spleen, NAD, slightly confused [illegible]
88 lbs, confused, no work
84 lbs, do, do

Date	Notes on the Cases
2.11.43	88 lbs, quiet, slightly confused, no work, good health
2.3.44	92 lbs, says he was selling Quaran but other point contradicts, excited for a minute, smiled, enjoyed the joke
	95 lbs, mentally same, no change, wants to go home
2.5.44	98 lbs, quiet
2.6.44	98 lbs, quiet
5.7.44	97 lbs, quiet
8.8.44	97 lbs, quiet
4.9.44	97 lbs, quiet, physical health, NAD
8.10.44	98 lbs, quiet, no work
3.11.44	96 lbs, quiet no work
8.12.44	97 lbs, quiet, no work
10.1.45	96 lbs, quiet
15.2.45	97 lbs, quiet, no work
16.3.45	96 lbs, quiet, no work
14.4.45	says that he was caught by [illegible] at 2 a.m. [illegible]
3.4.45	96 lbs, same, no change
13.5.45	98 lbs, quiet
6.7.45	94 lbs, quiet
2.9.45	98 lbs, do, no work
7.10.45	95 lbs, quiet, no work
14.11.45	98 lbs, quiet
6.12.45	98 lbs, do
13.12.45	does not do any work, still excited
12.1.46	96 lbs, obedient, no work
23.2.46	98 lbs, do, do
14.3.45	95 lbs, do, do
9.4.46	98 lbs, do, do
8.5.46	100 lbs, do, do
5.6.46	102 lbs, do, do
5.7.46	100 lbs, do, do
9.8.46	102 lbs, do, do
9.9.46	102 lbs, do, do
22.10.46	102 lbs, working in WS compound

Date	Notes on the Cases
2.11.46	102 lbs, do, do
4.12.46	102 lbs, quiet in working in WS compound
7.2.47	98 lbs
4.3.47	98 lbs, he does not work
8.4.47	98 lbs, no work
6.5.47	98 lbs, no work
3.6.47	99 lbs, no work
5.7.47	104 lbs, no work
2.8.47	102 lbs, no work
15.2.47	he has suppressed much and wants to go home

Appendix 3

Name- Bachu Lal alias Bachu Ram s/o Lachi Singh alias Lachi Ram	**Age-** 28
Caste- Thakur	**Occupation-**
Received from- Benares M. H.	**Date of Admission-** 16.9.38
Mental Disease- N.A.D.	**Cause-**
Date of Discharge- 21.11.38	**Result of Treatment-** Otherwise
Health on Admission- Fair	**Weight-** 112
Health on Discharge- Good	**Weight-** 122
Residence- No Relatives Nainital	**Vaccination-** Long scar behind right knee joint, one scar on the left foot, vaccinated

Copy of the Certificate- that he abused prisoners, had disrespectful conduct, sometimes talk sensibly, sometimes irrelevant, sometimes did answers questions and sometimes made certain peculiar bodily movements and sometimes refused food drink and changes of clothing, sometimes sang, gets excited at trifling affairs, speaking of high ideas & high people whom he probably does not know, sometimes found walking briskly inside the cells.

Signed
R.N. Bhandari
Supd., Central Jail
Allahabad

Date	Notes on the Cases
27.4.33	Committed a dacoity with deadly weapons at a bank at Ootacamund with 4 and 5 other terrorists
7.7.33	Sentenced to transportation for life (25 years) but the sentence was reduced to 10 years rigorous imprisonment on appeal in Coimbatore
26.1.34	arrived at Port Blair
8.2.36	assaulted a deputy jailor in Andaman
15.5.36	went on hunger strike from 15.5.36 to 18.5.36
29.8.36	burnt govt. clothing
22.9.37	left Port Blair
30.9.3	arrived at Naini central prison
18.9.37	promoted to B class
27.10.37	transferred to Benares Mental Hospital
22.12.37	kicked hospital attendant
10.6.38	tore up bed sheets
16.9.38	arrived at Agra Mental Hospital
13.9.38	defiant supercilious attitude, adding he is not a dacoit but was working in halwais shop in Amritsar before his arrest

Violent and dangerous, warn staff, possibly suicidal

16.9.38	Had a rag plug in his urthera
	Lungs, not adventitious sound

Date	Notes on the Cases
	Heart, not enlarged no murmur
	Spleen, not enlarged
	Liver, not enlarged

Ringworm around the waist

Date	Notes on the Cases
16.9.38	ringworm ointment prescribed for ringworm
16.9.38	made a false complaint that he was assaulted by the gatekeeper on arrival from Benares
24.9.38	up to the last night he was sleeping on bed which was given to him but tonight refused to sleep on the bed and slept on the floor. This morning he complained to the superintendent that the 2nd and 3rd class patients should be searched and particularly he should not be searched
5.10.38	a sharp piece of iron was found with his possession at the time of locking when he was searched. He became violent at the time and kicked attendant Jafail Ahmad. He also rushed on other patients but was prevented by other attendants on duty
6.10.38	a small piece of glass was found in his possession at the time of lock-up last evening
7.10.38	noisy and demonstrative, threatens to go on hunger strike
16.10.38	sensible, no work
17.10.38	saw the district judge and said that he did not like being kept under restraint
18.10.38	a new blanket coat was supplied to him yesterday but he refused to wear it and said it is too large for him
5.11.38	122 lbs, sensible, no work

Discharged under Section 31
21.11.38

Appendix 4

Name- Baijnath S/o Kundan	**Age-** 32
Caste- Ahir	**Occupation-**
Received from- Agra	**Date of Admission-** 29.4.38
Mental Disease- Schizophrenia	**Cause-**
Date of Discharge- 26.3.42	**Result of Treatment-** Cured
Health on Admission- Fair	**Weight-** 94 lbs
Health on Discharge- Fair	**Weight-** 100 lbs
Residence- Fyzabad Cant.	**Marks of Identification-** One mole left ankle, one scar laterally on left spine [illegible]
Vaccination- Not vaccinated	

Copy of Medical Certificate- Aggressive, claims to be khilafat worker and law breaker, refuses food: uncontrollable

Signed
Dr B. Das
Superintendent Mental Hospital Agra

Date	Notes on the Cases
30.4.38	Pyorrhea, to see dentist
	Lungs, not adventitious sound
	Heart, not enlarged no murmur
	Spleen, not enlarged
	Liver, not enlarged
8.5.38	92 lbs, confused, cleaning
1.5.38	vaccinated
7.6.38	98 lbs, incoherent, do
7.7.38	92 lbs, irrelevant, cleaning
7.7.38	100 lbs, confused, no work, got dysentery, admitted
7.9.38	96 lbs, incoherent, cleaning
10.10.38	96 lbs, dull, do
5.11.38	96 lbs, sensible, do
7.12.38	97 lbs, sensible, do
4.1.39	90 lbs, sensible, no, work, no physical ailment
11.1.39	90 lbs, he struck patient Mattri on his head
7.2.39	94 lbs, excitable, no work
8.3.39	92 lbs, irritable, no work
9.4.39	94 lbs, confused, do
10.5.39	96 lbs, irritable, do
11.6.39	95 lbs, sensible, do
7.7.39	92 lbs, sensible, do
11.6.39	95 lbs, sensible, do
7.7.39	92 lbs, sensible, do
9.8.39	90 lbs, sensible, do
10.9.39	90 lbs, sensible, do
11.11.39	95 lbs, sensible, do
11.12.39	97 lbs, incoherent, do

Date	Notes on the Cases
1.1.40	97 lbs, excitable, no physical work
1.2.40	99 lbs, not sensible
10.3.40	96 lbs
16.4.40	100 lbs, incoherent
6.5.40	98 lbs, quiet, height 5'2.5
8.6.40	100 lbs, incoherent
7.7.40	98 lbs, quiet
8.8.40	100 lbs, incoherent
7.9.40	98 lbs, quiet
8.10.40	100 lbs, quiet
14.11.40	100 lbs, sensible
15.12.40	100 lbs, sensible
5.1.41	101 lbs, quiet
8.2.41	100 lbs, quiet

[The case notes of the patient from 8.2.41 to 26.3.42 (that is, cured/discharged) are missing.]

Appendix 5

Name- Khanshah & Abdul Rahaman   **Age-** 55
     S/o Haji Gulam Husain

Caste- Muslim   **Occupation-** Contractor

Received from- Roorki   **Date of Admission-** 9.8.38

Mental Disease- N.A.D.   **Cause-**
     [Paranoid was replaced with N.A.D.
     in the case register].

Discharge of Treatment- 26.12.38   **Result of Treatment-**
                                         Otherwise

Health on Admission- Bad   **Weight-** 135 lbs

Health on Discharge- Good   **Weight-** 150 lbs

Residence- Sons Habib Rahman & Mohd Yusuf, Saathi Roorke	**Vaccination-** Big burn scar on left foot near limb toe, scar on the left [illegible], vaccinated

Copy of Medical Certificate- He is suffering from delusions in that he stated that Congress wants to kill him that he has had instructions from God that he was to kill all Hindus who were congressmen; that an attempt was made on his life, when travelling to Sahranpur.

Dr Rizvi
Medical Officer
Civil Hospitals, Roorkee

The wheel of the car came off. This incident is known to be true but the patient stated that the Dr Rizvi attempted to kill him, while under observation he would only have one particular mohmmaden cook to prepare his meals as he stated that others were bringing poison to do away with him. He feared persecution from the chairman of municipality R S Muthura Dass and therefore ward off doors of his quarters. He petitioned that he should send for twelve strong men from Rampur state to murder and to act as his bodyguard. He also stated that R S Muthura Dass had turned his sons against him leading his third son congress doctrines. So that the son attacked him and beat him as the son was patient in the civil hospital, Roorkee. [illegible] Information given by the eldest son that father beats sons.

He intervened governor of UP on question of approaching government to lay down railway for Haji pilgrims in Persia and to make a complaint against SDO, Roorke for being in league and congress to put down Mohammad but states that he states that he has no fear as life is drawing to close—god has given him sufficient strength to kill all the Hindus.

Signed
John Ravens
Captain IMS
Roorke

Date	Notes on the Cases
10.8.38	reticent, refuses to talk says that he is free from mental trouble, has lost all teeth
10.8.38	no teeth Lungs, no adventitious sounds Heart, not enlarged no murmurs Spleen, not enlarged Lungs, not enlarged
7.9.38	140 lbs, sensible, BC
10.10.38	144 lbs, do
14.10.38	no teeth, no physical ailment
5.11.38	140 lbs, sensible, no work
21.11.38	interviewed by Mohd. Yusuf son-in-law in my presence, explained all incidents, but admitted slapping sweeper as he lost his temper, refuses to go to Roorkee
7.12.38	150 lbs, sensible, reads books

Discharged under section 31
26.12.38

Appendix 6

Name- Raghu Nath Rai S/o Basu Rai	**Age-** 50
Caste- Hindu	**Occupation-** Zamindar
Received from- Ghazipur	**Date of Admission-** 21.8.38
Mental Disease- Dementia	**Cause-** old age
Date of Discharge- 24.1.39	**Result of Treatment-** Died
Health on Admission- Bad	**Weight-**
Health on Discharge-	**Weight-** 110 lbs
Residence- Shivo Devi Rai Joga Musahib Karimuddinpur, Ghazipur	**Marks of Identification-** Enlarged gland (cyst), [illegible] right side upper lip. One scar right [illegible], one mole on right calf
Vaccination- vaccinated	

Copy of the Medical Certificate- is violent and abusive, dirty in habits, remains naked, tears his clothes. Has damaged the walls of the cell badly under the impulse of insanity, sleeps and eats sparingly

Signed [illegible]
Supd. Dist. Jail
Ghazipur

Date	Notes on the Cases
22.8.38	Pyorrhoea, to see dentist
	Lungs, not adventitious sound
	Heart, not enlarged, no murmur
	Spleen, not enlarged
	Liver, not enlarged
7.9.38	110 lbs, dull, no work
10.10.38	114 lbs, excited, do
5.11.38	114 lbs, dementia, no work
5.12.38	111 lbs, dull, do
4.1.39	102 lbs, excited no physical ailment, except in abscesses on right elbow
7.1.39	very much excited, bromide mix, BO
11.1.39	abscess of [sic] opened by Deputy Superintendent and dressed antiseptically

Died of maniacal excitement
24.1.39

Appendix 7

Name- S. N. Ray	**Age-** 50 years
Caste- Brahmin	**Occupation-** Lecturer in physics
Received from- Lucknow	**Date of Admission-** 12.1.37
Mental Disease- Paranoid Dementia	**Cause-** Previous attack
Result of Treatment- Expired 15.12.51 at 5 a.m.	**Health on Admission-** Fair
Weight- 114 lbs	**Health on Discharge-**
Weight-	**Residence-**
Vaccination	

Date	Notes on the Cases
8.8.46	88 lbs, he was at infirmary for dysentery, no work
8.9.46	90 lbs, excited and destructive, no work
20.10.46	90 lbs, he was in infirmary for dysentery. He is improving now.
10.11.46	90 lbs
2. 12.46	90 lbs, he is now improving. He has torn all his clothing. He is at times very obstinate
8.1.47	94 lbs, he has gained weight, he is very destructive, he has torn most of his clothing given to him recently by Mrs. Ray
7.2.47	100 lbs
8.3.47	101 lbs, he does no work, sleeps and eats well
18.3.47	102 lbs, he was beaten by Jasbeer Singh after he quarrelled with him
6.4.47	His general health maintained. No change in his mental condition and habits (tears clothes)
25.5.47	He got excited and beat Ram Narain attendant
13.6.47	[illegible] 98 lbs, sulfosin, he has shown no improvement, his general health maintained
6.7.47	94 lbs, mentally shown no improvement, appetite less than before. At times he gets excited and inflicts injury to the other inmates of the hospital or the attendants
4.8.47	102 lbs, gained in physical health. Mentally he is just the same
6.9.47	104 lbs, physical health maintained. Mental condition same. Nowadays he does not get sleep at night
6.10.47	100 lbs, during the month of September he was excited now and then. Tears his clothing. Poor sleep.
14.10.47	Stool Examination [illegible]
1.11.47	100 lbs, physical health maintained. He tears all the beddings (blanket and dari). He at times is very excited. Violent, abusive, remains absolutely naked. Sometimes in the day and often at night
7. 12.47	98 lbs, confused and incoherent

Date	Notes on the Cases
15.1.48	His general health maintained. At times he becomes violent and abusive. His habit of tearing clothes is unavoidable.
1.3.48	99 lbs, incoherent. Roams around aimlessly. On being asked what work he does he said he tears garment. Roams around aimlessly. Destructive. No work Stool examination, cyst + roc++
16.4.48	97 lbs, same as before. He was suffering of ametoic dysentery from 10.4.48. [illegible] proper treatment given. He is now doing well but physical health is poor.

[Date of recorded treatment not clear]

	remains mostly agitated, destructive, eats well, sleeps well, E.S. therapy has been starts [*sic*] on 25.8.48, inconsequential talks, physical health maintained
11.10.48	not weighted
17.11.48	102 lbs, mentally same as before
14.12.48	patient is alright with ECT. If the periods are prolonged, he gets bad. He was excited on 9th, indecent and bad. He torn his shirt

ECT Record 25.8.48 to 27.10.48, 21 shocks biweekly and seven daily. Restrarted at 19.11.48 patient has received 7 shocks up to 13.12.48

Keeps manageable when he is getting electricity otherwise he is very destructive and mischievous

3.1.49	106 lbs
3.2.49	Mental condition as same

[The case notes between the period of 3.2.49 to 11.50 are missing.]

11.50	he is doing well. He cannot tolerate if some patient remarks or rebukes him. He then hits blindly otherwise. He is behaving well. Still makes best use of pieces of clothes. He is not picking of weight from last three months [illegible]

Date	Notes on the Cases
23.1.51	96 lbs
20.2.51	96 lbs
20.3.51	96 lbs
15.4.51	mentally he is just the same. At times he gets excited and quarrels other patient [*sic*]. He often tries to attack them also. He often tears off his clothes. His general health is fair.
26.4.51	100 lbs
25.5.51	97 lbs
10.7.51	no change in his mental condition. Dresses himself sometimes normally. Gets irritable very easily. Eats and sleep well.
26.8.51	*mera record dekh lijiye. Kabhi seeti nahin bajaiye. Shashra aur shastriyat chulah mein jaye. Hum nahin padhiyege, dusre padiyege. Sirf physics padhoga. Gomti par jaana palunga aur machli pakarunga.* He tears off his clothes and sleeps well. His physical poor. Weight 88 lbs. He takes 2, 3 chapatis but eats rice well. ECT Anaemic [illegible]
30.8.51	91 lbs
11.9.51	he had diarrhea, weakness and anemia and was transferred to infirmary on 28.8.51, he eats and sleeps well. Answers the question and talks irrelevantly
20.9.51	90 lbs, he again have a rise in temp [*sic*]. Since the 13th September going between [illegible] to 100 F, he was given thrymrol course for HW infection in Sept. He sleeps well up to 9 to 8 hours. Health is weak.
30.9.51	90 lbs He is weak and anaemic. His B.P is 139/52. He is again becoming destructive as he has started taking off his clothes. He talks irrelevant
2.11.51	90 lbs, he was having a little rise of temp daily in the evening for which he was fully investigated. Widal reaction negative. Urine culture also negative. He suffers from secondary by podoromic anaemic, stool examination negative

Date	Notes on the Cases
5.11.51	89 lbs
7.11.51	increased differently in [illegible]
11.11.51	temp 100 F
14.11.51	he is highly excited and gets angry on trifle
23.11.51	mitral regulation, murmur present, slight redness in feet [illegible] cough
27.11.51	Dr Mathur says he is a case of mitral [illegible]
28.11.51	
30.11.51	marked redness of feet and puffiness of feet
7.12.51	general debility, pulse between 109×110 marked [illegible]. Both heart murmur replaces murmur in mitral area
14.12.51	pulse irregular. Feeble
15.12.51	gradually weakening, pulse gradually missing and becoming weaker

Expired at 5. a.m. 15.12.51

Appendix 8

Name- Ismail Khan

Caste- Muslim

Received from- Agra

Mental Disease- Melancholia

Date of Discharge- 18.6.40

Health on Admission- Fair

Health on Discharge- Good

Residence- Ghaziabad, Meerut

Vaccination- not vaccinated,
    vaccinated 26.3.38

Age- 35

Occupation- Railway Service

Date of Admission- 30.3.38

Cause-

Result of Treatment- Improved

Weight- 98 lbs

Weigh- 107

Marks of Identification-
    One Mole on Left Ear, One
    Scar on Right Leg

Copy of Medical Certificate- Has delusions of having committed unpardonable sins, of having insulted great men, dull, and depressed Suicidal

Signed
Dr. B. Das
Superintendent Mental Hospital, Agra

Relatives/friends visit
9/9/38 Asst MO East India Railway Tundla
4/12/39, E.I Railway, Tundla Loco [illegible]

Date	Notes on the Cases
31.3.38	Pyorrhea, to see dentist
	Lungs, not adventitious sound
	Heart, not enlarged no murmur
	Spleen, not enlarged
	Liver, not enlarged
7.4.38	90 lbs, depressed, cleaning
2.5.38	Inquiry Nannhy Khan Driver Block (96)
	E I R Tundla
8.5.38	102 lbs, quiet, cleaning
1.5.38	vaccinated
7.6.38	106 lbs, depressed, factory
7.7.38	110 lbs, dull, factory
1.8.38	114 lbs, sensible, factory
7.9.38	110 lbs, incoherent, do
10.10.38	108 lbs, sensible, do
5.11.38	106 lbs, sensible, do
7.12.38	108 lbs, depressed, do
4.1.38	106 lbs, sensible, factory, no physical ailment
7.2.39	100 lbs, depressed, do
8.3.39	104 lbs, confused, do
9.4.39	104 lbs, quiet, do
10.5.39	102 lbs, depressed, do
11.6.39	102 lbs, confused, do

Date	Notes on the Cases
7.7.39	98 lbs, quiet, do
9.8.39	104 lbs, confused, do
10.9.39	103 lbs, depressed, do
10.10.39	103 lbs, dull, do
11.11.39	102 lbs, quiet, do
11.12.39	102 lbs, depressed, no physical ailment
8.1.40	104 lbs, depressed, brick making
8.2.40	104 lbs, better than before
5.3.40	104 lbs, quiet
16.4.40	104 lbs, better than before
10.5.40	104 lbs
11.6.40	105 lbs, improving
18.6.40	Discharged Under Section 33

Appendix 9

Name- Gopal Narian s/o Rudra Narian	**Age-** 18 yrs
Caste- Kayasth	**Occupation-** Student
Received from- Agra	**Date of Admission-** 3.9.38
Mental Disease- Confusional Insanity	**Cause-** Business Worry
Date of Discharge- 30.6.39	**Result of Treatment-** Otherwise
Health on Admission- Fair	**Weight-** 145 lbs
Health on Discharge- Good	**Weight-** 145 lbs
Residence- Cousin Bal Krishana alias Lalla dogawan near Hazrat B. Gunj, Bhadar alias Rambabu, Lucknow.	**Marks of identification-** Two moles on the neck, one scar on the right eye, one mole on the right middle finger
Vaccination- Vaccinated	

Copy of Medical Certificate- Explosive, excitable, wants to marry Kamla Jharia famous radio singer, has grandious [*sic*] ideas about himself.

Signature

Dr. B. Das

Supd. Mental Hospital Agra

[Additional information is given regarding family]

3.9.38

Late Rudra Narain Vakil

Dogoan, Lucknow

Sahj Ram Advocate

Zelia ganj, Lucknow

Date	Notes on the Cases
5.9.38	Lungs not adventitious sound
	Heart not enlarged, no murmur
	Spleen not enlarged
	Liver not enlarged
	112

[Additional information is given, Hospital visitation]
Balkrishna C/o K. B. Agarvala and Sons
                    2A Aminabad & sons
                    Lucknow

5.11.38	120 lbs, sensible, BC
7.12.38	125 lbs, sensible, do
4.1.39	130 lbs, sensible, no physical ailment
7.2.39	135 lbs, sensible, do
8.3.39	140 lbs, sensible, BC
9.4.39	140 lbs, sensible, BC
5.5.39	140 lbs, sensible, BC
8.6.39	145 lbs, quite sensible
30.6.39	discharged under S 32

Appendix 10

Name- Palhoo s/o Ghulam	**Age-** 26 yrs
Caste- Mohd	**Occupation-** Cultivator
Received from – Basirpur village ... Montgomery	**Date of Admission-** 19.12.1930
Mental Disease- Post, encephalitis	**Cause-** Infection
Date of Discharge- Died 13.12.47	**Result of Treatment-**
Health on Admission-	**Weight-** 130 lbs
Health on Discharge- Not Applicable	**Residence-** Basirpur ... Montogomery
Marks of identification-	**Vaccination-**

Copy of Medical Certificate- Talks incoherently and unintelligently. Dirty is his habits, takes food etc. Looks very unintelligent. does not ask questions properly. Behaves like a lunatic.

Major S. D. Sondhi
IMS Superintendent of Jail
Montgomery

+ Convicted of the offence of thefts of a coat with Railway badges and buttons, under section 379/75 of I.P.C and was sentenced to eighteen months of rigorous imprisonment including one month of solitary confinement. Talks incoherently and unintelligently, dirty is his habits, takes food etc. Looks very unintelligent. does not ask questions properly. Behaves like a lunatic.

+ Patient was convicted for stealing a coat and sentenced to 18 months imprisonment. He is a foolish looking man who talks indistinctly but sensibly. States that he is married and has one son about 3 year old. Was in form. Admits his crime. Memory is fair and good. Is ... both to time or place. does not seem to suffer from any hallucination or delusion. Can answer simple facts but does not know how many pice are there in 12 annas. Cannot count beyond 30. Appears to be feeble minded. Is shaky. Gait appears to be a little unsteady. There is a slight rigidity of ... but no definite ... Habits are clean, is well behaved and obedient, has his food, reads well.

Date	Notes on the Cases
26.12.30	repeats over and over again that he is sane, well behaved, and obedient
2.1.31	134 lbs, always stealing others' things
2.2.31	132 lbs, same
2.2.31	132 lbs, a very troublesome patient, teases others, steals other patients' things.
4.5.31	132 lbs, has vacant looks, mischievous, eats and sleeps well
2.6.31	130 lbs, keeping fit
10.3.31	126 lbs, keeping fit

Date	Notes on the Cases
5.8.31	124 lbs, keeping fit
8.9.31	124 lbs, mentally is bad
6.10.31	128 lbs, same
7.11.31	128 lbs, very mischievous
10.12.31	130 lbs, same
5.1.32	126 lbs, in hospital, teases others
3.2.32	128 lbs, is ill in the hospital, with gonorrhoea
11.3.32	129 lbs, repeats the same answer several times
2.4.32	128 lbs, same
3.5.32	124 lbs, repeats automatically the same sentence, so mischievous
2.6.32	122 lbs, no change
5.7.32	116 lbs, steals things, repeats the same sentence automatically post encephalitis
4.8.32	124 lbs, same
5.9.32	124 lbs, post encephalitis, repeats the same words several times, mischievous
7.10.32	126 lbs, no change
6.11.32	126 lbs, no change
5.12.32	126 lbs, no change
19.1.33	122 lbs, affectionately embraces others, sodomist
10.2.33	128 lbs, emotional
9.3.33	124 lbs, same
25.4.33	126 lbs, dementia, emotional, wishes to go home. Works a little
13.5.33	126 lbs, no change
10.6.33	126 lbs, affectionately embraces others. Foolish. Desires to go home
11.9.33	126 lbs, do
10.8.33	122 lbs, no change
11.9.33	124 lbs, same
13.10.33	124 lbs, he is very mischievous and annoys other patients, repeats the same words post encephalitis, his statements are unreliable and changes them from time to time

Date	Notes on the Cases
13.11.33	125 lbs, same
6.12.33	125 lbs, same
12.1.34	123 lbs, same
10.2.34	122 lbs, same
10.3.34	122 lbs, same
9.4.34	122 lbs, same
7.5.34	122 lbs, same
9.6.34	123 lbs, assaulted patient, mischievous
7.7.34	122 lbs, he is very troublesome patient and tries to commit sodomy, post E.R.
16.8.34	122 lbs, same
11.9.34	122 lbs, same
10.10.34	122 lbs, same
8.11.34	125 lbs, same
14.12.34	127 lbs, same
19.1.35	128 lbs, same
19.3.35	122 lbs, he repeats the same word, his speech affected, post E.R. troublesome
29.4.35	127 lbs, dementia, sick: post encephalitic psychosis … mischievous
13.5.35	127 lbs, same
11.6.35	125 lbs, no change
3.7.35	125 lbs, same
5.8.35	125 lbs, same
7.4.35	125 lbs, same
7.9.35	126 lbs, same
10.10.35	123 lbs, tremor all over the body
5.11.35	126 lbs, same
6.12.35	125 lbs, same
11.1.36	126 lbs, same
5.2.36	126 lbs, same
10.3.36	125 lbs, same
14.4.36	124 lbs, same
8.5.36	125 lbs, same
14.4.36	124 lbs, same

Date	Notes on the Cases
8.5.36	118 lbs, same
5.6.36	120 lbs, same
4.7.36	120 lbs, same
7.8.36	121 lbs, same
5.9.36	121 lbs, same
5.10.36	124 lbs, same
7.11.36	121 lbs, same
8.12.36	121 lbs, same
13.1.37	124 lbs, same
14.02.37	124 lbs, same
5.3.1937	122 lbs, no improvement, dementia, embraces arms of the people
19.4.37	123 lbs, same
5.5.37	125 lbs, same
8.6.37	125 lbs, same
2.7.37	124 lbs, same
6.8.37	124 lbs, same
3.9.37	124 lbs, same
9.10.37	120 lbs, no change
9.11.37	121 lbs, same
8.12.37	129 lbs, same
6.1.38	128 lbs, same
2.3.38	128 lbs, same
7.3.38	124 lbs, same
8.4.38	126 lbs, same
7.5.38	122 lbs, same
14.6.38	122 lbs, no improvement
6.7.38	126 lbs, same
15.8.38	126 lbs, in hospital for a wound on the right hand. Mentally same
4.9.38	122 lbs, no improvement mentally
6.10.38	126 lbs, same
8.11.38	same, embraces people
6.12.38	126 lbs, same
7.1.39	123 lbs, same

Date	Notes on the Cases
21.2.39	130 lbs, same
7.3.39	127 lbs, same
17.4.39	130 lbs, same
18.5.39	128 lbs, same
9.6.39	126 lbs, same
11.7.39	127 lbs, same
3.8.39	120 lbs, same
7.10.39	125 lbs, same
7.11.39	124 lbs, same
16.12.39	124 lbs, sodomist, same
11.1.40	127 lbs, same, masturbates
10.2.40	131 lbs, same
11.3.40	130 lbs, sodomist, same, always lying down
13.4.40	131 lbs, same
13.5.40	132 lbs, same
19.6.40	126 lbs, same
16.7.40	128 lbs, same
12.8.40	132 lbs, same
8.9.40	131 lbs, no change
14.10.40	126 lbs, sexual pervert, tremors, flow of saliva constant, post encephalitic symptoms
22.11.40	129 lbs, same
22.12.40	128 lbs, same
23.1.41	129 lbs, no change. Gets epileptic attacks about twice a month, when he remains for the whole of the day semi-conscious, but can be roused by a loud call. Then he does not take food also.
17.2.41	128 lbs, epileptic attacks more frequent (4–5 in a month), to be transferred to old hospital section for observation
17.3.41	128 lbs, same
19.4.41	131 lbs, no change
19.5.41	130 lbs, same
20.6.41	130 lbs, no change
8.7.41	130 lbs, no change

Date	Notes on the Cases
16.8.41	126 lbs, very mischievous and sodomistic
8.9.41	127 lbs, same
11.10.41	127 lbs, same
12.11.41	no change
25.12.41	120 lbs, same
28.1.42	125 lbs, same
11.2.42	122 lbs, same
17.3.42	121 lbs, no change
24.4.42	122 lbs, same
21.5.42	122 lbs, no change
16.6.43	121 lbs, same
28.7.42	117 lbs, same
22.8.42	118 lbs, sexual pervert, post encephalitic, characteristic speech, tremors, saliva dribbles from his mouth, clean, helps in the section
22.9.42	115 lbs, same
16.10.42	113 lbs, same, hides articles, beats patients
18.11.42	114 lbs, no change
14.12.42	113 lbs, same
16.1.43	114 lbs, no change
19.2.43	116 lbs, same
12.3.43	115 lbs, same
10.4.43	112 lbs, same
19.6.43	110 lbs, same
13.7.43	110 lbs, has a septic ulcer on foot, same mentally
20.8.43	112 lbs, same
13.9.43	112 lbs, same
15.10.43	110 lbs, same
12.11.43	111 lbs, no change
11.12.43	113 lbs, same
12.1.44	118 lbs, no change, wants to go to his wife
10.2.44	121 lbs, same
16.3.44	118 lbs, same
11.4.44	122 lbs, same
17.5.44	118 lbs, no lice, same mentally

Date	Notes on the Cases
14.6.44	114 lbs, same as before
14.7.44	117 lbs, no lice, vaccinated against smallpox. Milk stopped and also gur stopped
16.8.44	114 lbs, no lice, same mentally
18.9.44	118 lbs, same as previously
26.10.44	117 lbs, no change, helps attendant
24.11.44	115 lbs, same
19.1.45	117 lbs, no change
20.2.45	122 lbs, same mentally
17.3.45	125 lbs, no change mentally. Improved.
28.4.45	122 lbs, same, sodomistic
25.5.45	118 lbs, no change
25.6.45	115 lbs, progressive loss of weight. Referred to Hospital. Extremely sodomistic. Always on the look-out to entice the demented for the purpose
17.7.45	116 lbs, same
23.9.45	109 lbs, referred to hospital for loss of weight. Same mentally
15.11.45	114 lbs, saliva dribbling from mouth
20.12.45	122 lbs, no change at all
20.2.46	122 lbs, same
20.2.46	120 lbs, same
16.3.46	122 lbs, no change
26.4.46	110 lbs, same
25.5.46	114 lbs, same
28.6.46	116 lbs, same
31.7.46	112 lbs, same
5.9.46	118 lbs, no change
17.10.46	114 lbs, same
22.11.46	118 lbs, no change
4.1.47	112 lbs, no change, deteriorating
2.2.47	110 lbs, not improving
10.3.47	same
6.4.47	ulcer on both lips, disorientated, obstinate
29.4.47	110 lbs, ulcers better, mentally same

Date	Notes on the Cases
31.5.47	110 lbs, same
29.6.47	111 lbs, same
28.7.47	112 lbs, same
30.8.47	110 lbs, same
8.10.47	108 lbs, same
8.11.47	in hospital

Died of general debility in ward today at 9.30 a.m.
13.12.47

Bibliography

Primary Sources

Archival Sources

Home Department/Jails Branch 1905–39
Home Department/Medical Branch 1862–1930
Home Department/Public Branch 1860–95
India Records, Nehru Memorial Museum and Library, Delhi
Medical Board Proceedings 1820–58
National Archives of India, New Delhi
Proceedings and Files of the Government of Punjab including the Public and
the Jail Branch. Punjab State Archives, Chandigarh
Proceedings to the Legislative Department 1860–1940
Unpublished Case Histories. Agra Mental Hospital Records, Agra
Unpublished Case Histories. Lahore Mental Hospital Records, Lahore

Published Reports

Report of the Health Survey and Development Committee. Delhi: Manager of Publication, 1946.

Report of the Indian Hemp Drugs Commission 1893–1894. Simla: Government Central Printing Office, 1894.

Private Papers

Lodge Patch, Charles J. 'Birth of a Hospital' (unpublished, typescript account of the mental hospital in Lahore). Private Papers, Mss Eur F544, British Library.

Papers of Edward Mapother. Treatment of Mental Disorder in India File, Royal Bethlem Hospital Archives, Kent, England.

Journals

Aarogya Vigyan
Ayurveda Vigyan
Indian Medical Gazette
Journal of Mental Sciences
Man

Books Published before 1947

Anonymous. *Naujawan Kyun Maarey Jaate Hain* (Why young men die?). Lahore: Anglo-Sanskrit Press Lahore, n.d.

Chevers, Norman. *A Manual of Medical Jurisprudence for Bengal and North-Western Provinces.* Calcutta: Bengal Military Orphan Press, 1856.

Clark, Sir James. *A Memoir of John Conolly; Comprising the Sketch of the Treatment of the Insane in Europe and America.* London: John Murray, 1869.

Conolly, John. *The Construction and Government of Lunatic Asylums and Hospitals for the Insane.* London: Churchill, 1847.

Crawford, D. G. *A History of the Indian Medical Service 1600–1913.* London: Thacker & Co., 1914.

Dehati Chikitsak, Part 2. Hamdard Publication, n.d.

Ewens, G. F. W. *Insanity in India: Its Symptoms and Diagnosis: With Reference to the Relation of Crime and Insanity.* Calcutta: Thacker, Spink & Co., 1908, reprinted in Memphis: General Books, 2009.

Fr. Leo, O. M. Cap. *Missionary Apostolate in the Punjab.* Mangalore: Codialbail Press, 1910.

Ghosh, Birendra Nath. *A Treatise on Hygiene and Public Health: With Special Reference to the Tropics*, 9th ed. Calcutta: Scientific Publishing, 1938.

Halliday, Andrew. *A General View of the Present State of Lunatics, and Lunatic Asylums, in Great Britain and Ireland, and in Some Other Kingdoms*. London: Thomas and George Underwood, 1827.

Harnamdas, Kavita. *Yovan Raksha*. Lahore: 1936.

Hill, Robert Gardiner. *Lunacy: Its Past and Its Present*. London: Longman, Green, 1870.

Indra, Pandit Ganeshdutt. *Swapnadosh Vigyan*. Kashi: Kailashnath Bhargav 'Amar', 1949.

Modi, Jaising P. *A Textbook of Medical Jurisprudence and Toxicology*. Bombay: N. M. Tripathi Ltd, 1945.

Nagar, Durgashankar. *Prana Chikitsa (Psycho-Therapy—Its Doctrine and Practice)*. Lucknow: Adhyaksha Ganga Fine Art Press, 1931.

Overbeck-Wright, Alaxender William. *Lunacy in India*. London: Bailliere, Tindall and Cox, 1921.

Patch, Charles J. Lodge. *A Critical Review of the Punjab Mental Hospitals from 1840–1930*. Lahore Record Office: Punjab Government, 1931.

Shaw, W. S. Jagoe. *A Clinical Handbook of Mental Diseases: For the Use of Students and Medical Practitioners in India*. Calcutta: Butterworth & Co., 1925.

Tuke, Samuel. *Description of the Retreat: An Institution Near York for Insane Persons of the Society of Friends*. York, England: W. Alexander, 1813.

Secondary Sources

Books

Alavi, Seema. *Islam and Healing: Loss and Recovery of an Indo-Muslim Medical Tradition, 1600–1900*. Palgrave Macmillan, 2008.

Alter, Joseph S. *Gandhi's Body: Sex, Diet, and the Politics of Nationalism*. Philadelphia: University of Pennsylvania Press, 2000.

———. *The Wrestler's Body: Identity and Ideology in North India*. Berkeley: University of California Press, 1992.

Arnold, David, ed. *Imperial Medicine and Indigenous Societies*. Manchester: Manchester University Press, 1988.

Attwell, Guy. *Refiguring Unani Tibb: Plural Healing in Late Colonial India*. Hyderabad: Orient Longman, 2007.

Bandopadhyay, Sekhar. *From Plassey to Partition: A History of Modern India*. New Delhi: Orient Blackswan, 2004.

Bayly, C. A. *Empire and Information: Intelligence Gathering and Social Communication in India, 1750–1870.* New Delhi: Cambridge University Press, 1999.

Berkenkotter, Carol. *Patient Tales: Case Histories and the Uses of Narrative in Psychiatry.* Columbia: The University of South Carolina Press, 2008.

Berrios, German E. *The History of Mental Symptoms: Descriptive Psychopathology since the Nineteenth Century.* Cambridge: Cambridge University Press, 1996.

Bewley, Thomas. *Madness to Mental Illness: A History of the Royal College of Psychiatrists.* London: The Royal College of Psychiatrists, 2008.

Bhattacharya, B. K. *Insanity and Criminal Law.* Calcutta: Eastern Law House Private Ltd, 1964.

Bhugra, Dinesh, ed. *Psychiatry and Religion: Context, Consensus and Controversies.* London: Routledge, 1996.

Bose, Sugata. *The Nation as Mother and Other Visions of Nationhood.* Gurgaon, Haryana: Penguin Viking, 2017.

Chakrabarty, Dipesh. *Provincializing Europe: Postcolonial Thought and Historical Difference.* Princeton: Princeton University Press, 2000.

Chatterjee, Partha. *The Nation and Its Fragments: Colonial and Postcolonial Histories.* Princeton Studies Princeton: Princeton University Press, 1993.

Cohen, Lawrence. *No Aging in India: Modernity, Senility and the Family.* New Delhi: Oxford University Press, 1998.

Cohn, Bernard. *Colonialism and Its Forms of Knowledge.* In *The Bernard Cohn Omnibus.* New Delhi: Oxford University Press, 2008.

Conrad, Peter, and Joseph W. Schneider. *Deviance and Medicalization: From Badness to Sickness.* Philadelphia, Temple University Press, 1993.

Crabtree, Adam. *From Mesmer to Freud: Magnetic Sleep and the Roots of Psychological Healing.* New Haven: Yale University Press, 1993.

Crossley, Nick. *Contesting Psychiatry: Social Movements in Mental Health.* London: Routledge, 2006.

Dain, Norman. *Clifford W. Beers: Advocate for the Insane.* Pittsburgh: University of Pittsburgh Press, 1980.

Dalmia, Vasudha. *The Nationalisation of Hindu Traditions: Bharatendu Harischandra and Nineteenth-Century Banaras.* Delhi: Oxford University Press, 1997.

Darnton, Robert. *Mesmerism and the End of the Enlightenment in France.* Cambridge: Harvard University Press, 1968.

Das, Debjani. *Houses of Madness: Insanity and Asylums of Bengal in Nineteenth-Century India.* New Delhi: Oxford University Press, 2015.

Das, Rahul Peter. *The Origin of the Life of a Human Being: Conception and the Female According to Ancient Medical and Sexological Literature.* Delhi: Motilal Banarsidass Publishers Private Limited, 2003.

Ernst, Waltraud. *Colonialism and Transnational Psychiatry: The Development of an Indian Mental Hospital in British India, c. 1925–1940*. London: Anthem Press, 2013.

———. *Mad Tales from the Raj: The European Insane in British India, 1800–1858*. London: Routledge, 1991.

———. *Plural Medicine, Traditions and Modernity, 1800–2000*. London: Routledge, 2002.

———, ed. *Work, Psychiatry and Society, c.1750–2015*. Manchester: Manchester University Press, 2016.

Fabrega Jr., Horacio. *History of Mental Illness in India: A Cultural Psychiatry Retrospective*. Delhi: Motilal Banarasidas, 2009.

Fanon, Frantz. *Black Skin, White Masks*, translated by Charles Lam Markmann. London: Pluto Press, 2008 (first published in French in 1952).

———. *The Wretched of the Earth*, translated by Constance Farrington. New York: Grove Press, 1963.

Fissell, Mary E. *Vernacular Bodies: The Politics of Reproduction in Early Modern England*. Oxford: Oxford University Press, 2004.

Foucault, Michel. *Abnormal: Lectures at College de France, 1974–75*, translated by Graham Burchell. New Delhi: Navayana, 2010.

———. *Discipline and Punish: The Birth of Prison*, translated by Alan Sheridan. New York: Vintage Book, 1995.

———. *Madness and Civilization: A History of Insanity in the Age of Reason*, translated by Richard Howard. London: Routledge, 2001.

Fuechtner, Veronika, Douglas E. Haynes, and Ryan M. Jones, eds. *A Global History of Sexual Science, 1880–1960*. California: University of California Press, 2018.

Gijswijt-Hofstra, Marijke, Harry Oosterhuis, Joost Vijselaar, and Hugh Freeman, eds. *Psychiatric Cultures Compared: Psychiatry and Mental Health Care in the Twentieth Century*. Amsterdam: Amsterdam University Press, 2005.

Glover, William J. *Making Lahore Modern: Constructing and Imagining a Colonial City*. Minneapolis: University of Minnesota Press, 2008.

Goffman, Erving. *Asylums: Essays on the Social Situation of Mental Patients and Other Inmates*. Chicago: Aldine, 1962.

Goldstein, Jan. *Console and Classify: The French Psychiatric Profession in the Nineteenth Century*. Chicago: University of Chicago Press, 2001.

Green, Nile. *Islam and the Army in Colonial India: Sepoy Religion in the Service of Empire*. Cambridge: Cambridge University Press, 2009.

Gupta, Charu. *Sexuality, Obscenity, Community: Women, Muslims and the Hindu Public in Colonial India*. New York: Palgrave, 2002.

Gupta, Partha Sarthi. *Power, Politics and the People: Studies in British Imperialism and Indian Nationalism*. New Delhi: Permanent Black, 2001.

Halliburton, Murphy. *Mudpacks and Prozac: Experiencing Ayurvedic, Biomedical and Religious Healing.* California: Left Coast Press, 2009.

Hartnack, Christiane. *Psychoanalysis in Colonial India.* New Delhi: Oxford University Press, 2001.

Jaffrelot, Christophe. *The Hindu Nationalist Movement and Indian Politics: 1925 to the 1990s.* London: Hurst & Company, 1996.

Jones, Kathleen. *Mental Health and Social Policy 1845–1959.* London: Routledge, 1960.

Jones, Kenneth. *Socio-Religious Reform Movements in British India.* Albany: State University of New York Press, 1992.

Joshi, Sanjay. *Fractured Modernity: Making of a Middle Class in Colonial North India.* New Delhi: Oxford University Press, 2001.

Jurgensmeyer, Mark. *Religion as Social Vision: The Movement against Untouchability in Twentieth Century Punjab.* Berkeley: University of California Press, 1982.

Kakar, Sudhir. *Shamans, Mystics, and Doctors: A Psychological Inquiry into India and its Healing Traditions.* Delhi: Oxford University Press, 1992.

Kolsky, Elizabeth. *Colonial Justice in British India.* New Delhi: Cambridge University Press, 2010.

Kumar, Deepak. *Science and the Raj: A Study of British India.* New Delhi: Oxford University Press, 2006.

Laqueur, Thomas. *Making Sex: Body and Gender from the Greeks to Freud.* Cambridge: Harvard University Press, 1990.

———. *Solitary Sex: A Cultural History of Masturbation.* New York: Zone Books, 2003.

Ludke, Alf. *The History of Everyday Life: Reconstructing Historical Experiences and Ways of Life.* Princeton: Princeton University Press, 1995.

Mahone, Sloan, and Megan Vaughan, eds. *Psychiatry and Colonialism.* New York: Palgrave Macmillan, 2007.

Malhotra, Anshu. *Gender, Caste and Religious Identities: Restructuring Class in Colonial Punjab.* New Delhi: Oxford University Press, 2002.

Manto, Saadat Hasan. 'For Freedom Sake.' In *Black Margins,* edited by Muhammad Umar Memon, translated into English by M. Asaduddin, 105–34. Katha: Oxford University Press, 2001.

Marland, Hilary. *Dangerous Motherhood: Insanity and Childbirth in Victorian Britain.* Basingstoke and New York: Palgrave Macmillan, 2004.

Mayo, Katherine. *Mother India,* edited and with an introduction by Mrinalini Sinha. Ann Arbor: University of Michigan Press, 2000, 1998.

McCulloch, Jock. *Colonial Psychiatry and 'the African Mind'.* Cambridge: Cambridge University Press, 1995.

Melling, Joseph, and Bill Forsythe. *The Politics of Madness: The State, Insanity and Society in England, 1845–1914.* London: Routledge, 2006.

Menon, Dilip. *Caste, Nationalism and Communism in Malabar.* Cambridge: Cambridge University Press, 1994.

Metcalf, Thomas R. *Ideologies of the Raj.* Cambridge: Cambridge University Press, 1995.

Mills, James H. *Cannabis Britannica: Empire, Trade, and Prohibition, 1800–1928.* Oxford: Oxford University Press, 2005.

———. *Madness, Cannabis and Colonialism: The 'Native-Only' Lunatic Asylums of British India, 1857–1900.* Basingstoke: Macmillan, 2000.

Mishra, Saurabh. *Pilgrimage, Politics and Pestilence: The Haj from the Indian Subcontinent, 1860–1920.* New Delhi: Oxford University Press, 2011.

Misra, B. B. *The Indian Middle Classes: Their Growth in Modern Times.* London: Oxford University Press, 1961.

Monroe, John Warne. *Laboratories of Faith: Mesmerism, Spiritism and Occultism in Modern France.* London: Cornell University Press, 2008.

Mukharji, Projit Bihari. *Nationalizing the Body: The Medical Market, Print and Daktari Medicine.* London: Anthem Press, 2009.

Nandy, Ashis. *The Intimate Enemy: Loss and Recovery of Self under Colonialism.* Delhi: Oxford University Press, 1983.

———. *The Savage Freud and Other Essays on Possible and Retrievable Selves.* Princeton: Princeton University Press, 1995.

Pande, Ishita. *Medicine, Race and Liberalism in British Bengal: Symptoms of Empire.* London: Routledge, 2010.

Parry-Jones, William LI. *The Trade in Lunacy: A Study of Private Madhouses in England in the Eighteenth and Nineteenth Centuries.* London: Routledge & Kegan Paul, 1972.

Pati, Biswamoy, and Mark Harrison, eds. *The Social History of Health and Medicine in Colonial India.* London: Routledge, 2009.

———, eds. *Society, Medicine and Politics in Colonial India.* New Delhi: Routledge, 2018.

Pinch, William R. *Peasants and Monks in British India.* Berkeley: University of California Press, 1996.

———. *Warrior Ascetics and Indian Empires.* Cambridge: Cambridge University Press, 2006.

Pinto, Sarah. *Daughters of Parvati: Women and Madness in Contemporary India.* Philadelphia: University of Pennsylvania Press, 2014.

Porter, Roy. *Health for Sale: Quackery in England 1660–1850.* Manchester: Manchester University Press, 1989.

———. *Madness: A Brief History.* Oxford: Oxford University Press, 2002.

Porter, Roy, and David Wright, eds. *The Confinement of Insane: International Perspectives 1800–1965*. Cambridge: Cambridge University Press, 2003.

Prasad, Vijay. *Untouchable Freedom: A Social History of a Dalit Community*. New Delhi: Oxford University Press, 2000.

Radhakrishna, Meena. *Dishonoured by History: 'Criminal Tribes' and British Colonial Policy*. Hyderabad: Orient Longman, 2001.

Ripa, Yannick. *Women and Madness: The Incarceration of Women in Nineteenth Century France*. Cambridge: Polity Press, 1990.

Robinson, Francis. *Separatism among Indian Muslims: The Politics of the UP Muslims, 1860–1923*. Delhi: Oxford India Paperbacks, 1993.

Roelcke, Volker, Paul J. Weindling, and Louise Westwood, eds. *International Relations in Psychiatry: Britain, Germany, & The United States to World War II*. Rochester, NY; Woodbridge: University of Rochester Press, 2010.

Roper, Lynda. *Oedipus & the Devil: Witchcraft, Sexuality and Religion in Early Modern Europe*. London: Routledge, 1994.

Roy, Kumkum. *The Power of Gender and the Gender of Power: Explorations in Early Indian History*. New Delhi: Oxford University Press, 2010.

Sarkar, Sumit. *Modern India: 1885–1947*. Delhi: Macmillan India, 1983.

Sarkar, Tanika. *Hindu Wife, Hindu Nation: Community, Religion and Cultural Nationalism*. Delhi: Permanent Black, 2001.

Scull, Andrew. *Hysteria: The Disturbing History*. Oxford: Oxford University Press, 2009.

———. *The Most Solitary of Afflictions: Madness and Society in Britain, 1700–1900*. New Haven and London: Yale University Press, 1993.

Sharma, Madhuri. *Indigenous and Western Medicine in Colonial India*. New Delhi: Foundation Books, 2012.

Shorter, Edward. *A History of Psychiatry: From the Era of the Asylum to the Age of Prozac*. New York: John Wiley & Sons, 1997.

Showalter, Elaine. *The Female Malady: Women, Madness and English Culture, 1830–1980*. London: Virago Press, 1987.

Singha, Radhika. *A Despotism of Law: Crime and Justice in Early Colonial India*. New Delhi: Oxford University Press, 2000.

Sinha, Mrinalini. *Colonial Masculinity: The 'Manly Englishman' and the 'Effeminate Bengali' in the Late Nineteenth Century*. New York: Manchester University Press, 1995.

Sivaramakrishnan, Kavita. *Old Potions, New Bottles: Recasting Indigenous Medicine in Colonial Punjab, 1850–1945*. Hyderabad: Orient Longman, 2006.

Skultans, Vieda. *English Madness: Ideas on Insanity, 1580–1890*. London: Routledge, 1979.

Smith, Leonard D. *'Cure, Comfort and Safe Custody': Public Lunatic Asylums in Early Nineteenth-Century England.* London: Leicester University Press, 1999.

Suzuki, Akihito. *Madness at Home: The Psychiatrist, the Patient and the Family in England, 1820–1860.* California: University of California Press, 2006.

Tomlinson, B. R. *The Economy of Modern India 1860–1947.* Cambridge: Cambridge University Press, 1993.

Topp, Leslie., James E. Moran, and Jonathan Andrews, eds. *Madness, Architecture and the Built Environment.* London: Routledge, 2007.

Van Driel, Mels. *Manhood: The Rise and Fall of the Penis.* London: Reaktion Books, 2009.

Vanita, Ruth, and Saleem Kidwai, eds. *Same Sex Love in India.* New York: Palgrave Macmillan, 2000.

Vaughan, Megan. *Curing Their Ills: Colonial Power and African Illness.* Palo Alto: Stanford University Press, 1991.

Walsh, Judith E. *Domesticity in Colonial India What Women Learned When Men Gave Them Advice.* New York: Rowman and Littlefield Publishers, 2004.

———. *How to Be the Goddess of Your Home: An Anthology of Bengali Domestic Manuals.* New Delhi: Yoda Press, 2005.

Winterbottom, Anna, and Facil Tesfaye, eds. *Histories of Medicine and Healing in the Indian Ocean World,* vol. 1. London: Palgrave Macmillan, 2016.

White, David Gordon. *Sinister Yogis.* Chicago: University of Chicago Press, 2009.

Wright, David. *Mental Disability in Victorian England, the Earlswood Asylum, 1847–1901.* Oxford: Oxford University Press, 2001.

Wolfram, Heather. *The Stepchildren of Science, Psychical Research and Parapsychology in Germany, c. 1870–1939.* Amsterdam: Rodopi, 2009.

Chapters in Books

Ali, Daud. 'Aristocratic Body Techniques in Early Medieval India'. In *Rethinking a Millennium,* edited by Rajat Dutta. Delhi: Aakar Books, 2008.

Arnold, David. 'Vagrant India: Famine, Poverty and Welfare under Colonial Rule'. In *Cast Out: Vagrancy and Homelessness in Global and Historical Perspective,* edited by A. L. Beier and Paul Ocobock, 117–39. Ohio: Ohio University Press, 2008.

Cooter, Roger. 'Medicine and Modernity'. In *The Oxford Handbook of the History of Medicine,* edited by Mark Jackson, 100–16. Oxford: Oxford University Press, 2011.

Deacon, Harriet. 'Robben Island Lunatic Asylum, South Africa, 1846–1910'. In *The Confinement of Insane: International Perspectives 1800–1965*, edited by Roy Porter and David Wright, 20–53. Cambridge: Cambridge University Press, 2003.

Ernst, Waltraud. 'The Establishment of "Native Lunatic Asylums" in Early Nineteenth-Century British India'. In *Studies in Indian Medical History*, edited by G. Jan Meulenbeld and Dominik Wujastyk, 169–204. Delhi: Motilal Banarsidass, 2001.

———. 'Feminising Madness—Feminising the Orient: Gender, Madness and Colonialism, c. 1860–1940'. In *Exploring Gender: Colonial and Post-colonial India*, edited by S. Kak and B. Pati, 57–92. New Delhi: Nehru Memorial and Museum Library, 2005.

———. 'Madness and Colonial Spaces: British India, c. 1800–1947'. In *Madness, Architecture and the Built Environment*, edited by Leslie Topp, James Moran, and Jonathan Andrews. London: Routledge, 2007.

———. 'Out of Sight and Out of Mind: Insanity in Early Nineteenth Century India'. In *Insanity, Institutions and Society, 1800–1914: A Social History of Madness in Comparative Perspective*, edited by Joseph Melling and Bill Forsythe, 245–67. London: Routledge, 1999.

———. 'Practising "Colonial" Or "Modern" Psychiatry in British India? Treatments at the Indian Mental Hospital at Ranchi, 1925–1940'. In *Transnational Psychiatries: Social and Cultural Histories of Psychiatry in Comparative Perspective c. 1800–2000*, edited by Waltraud Ernst and Thomas Mueller, 80–115. Newcastle: Cambridge Scholars Publishing, 2010.

Gupta, Charu. 'Hindu Wombs, Muslim Progeny: The Numbers Game and Shifting Debates on Widow Remarriage in Uttar Pradesh, 1890s–1930s'. In *Reproductive Health in India History, Politics, Controversies*, edited by Sarah Hodges, 167–98. Hyderabad: Orient Longman Private Ltd, 2006.

Hodges, Sarah. 'Towards a History of Reproduction in Modern India'. In *Reproductive Health in India History, Politics, Controversies*, edited by Sarah Hodges, 1–21. Hyderabad: Orient Longman Private Ltd, 2006.

Lal, Maneesha. 'Purdah as Pathology: Gender and the Circulation of Medical Knowledge in Late Colonial India'. In *Reproductive Health in India History, Politics, Controversies*, edited by Sarah Hodges, 85–114. Hyderabad: Orient Longman Private Ltd, 2006.

Littlewood, Roland. 'Colonialism and Psychiatry'. In *Colonialism and Psychiatry*, edited by Dinesh Bhugra and Roland Littlewood, 1–14. New Delhi: Oxford University Press, 2002.

MacKinnon, Dolly. '"Amusements Are Provided": Asylum Entertainment and Recreation in Australia and New Zealand c.1860–c.1945'. In *Permeable Walls: Historical Perspectives on Hospital and Asylum Visiting*, edited by

Graham Mooney and Jonathan Reinarz, 267–88. New York: Rodopi, 2009.

Mills, James H. "'More Important to Civilize Than Subdue'? Lunatic Asylums, Psychiatric Practice and Fantasies of "the Civilizing Mission" in British India, 1858–1900'. In *Colonialism as a Civilizing Mission: Cultural Ideology in British India*', edited by Harald Fischer-Tine and Michael Mann, 179–90. London: Anthem South Asian Studies, 2004.

Mills, James H., and Patricia T. Barton. 'Introduction'. In *Drugs and Empire: Essays in Modern Imperialism and Intoxication, c. 1500–1930*, edited by James H. Mills and Patricia Barton, 1–16. New York: Palgrave Macmillan, 2007.

Padoux, Andre. 'What Do We Mean by Tantrism'. In *The Roots of Tantra*, edited by Katherine Anne Harper and Robert L. Brown. New York: State University of New York Press, 2002.

Persaud, Anil. 'Transformed Over Seas: "Medical Comforts" aboard Nineteenth-Century Emigrant Ships'. In *Labour Matters towards Global Histories*, edited by Marcel Van Der Linden and Prabhu P. Mahopatra, 22–56. New Delhi: Tulika Books, 2009.

Porter, Roy. 'The Body and the Mind, the Doctor and the Patient: Negotiating Hysteria'. In *Hysteria beyond Freud*, edited by Sander L. Gilman, Helen King, et al. Berkley: University of California Press, 2003.

Radhakrishna, Meena. 'Laws of Metamorphosis: From Nomad to Offender'. In *Challenging the Rule(s) of Law: Colonialism, Criminology and Human Rights in India*, edited by Kalpana Kannabiran and Ranbir Singh, 3–27. New Delhi: Sage, 2009.

Sarkar, Sumit. 'The "Women's Question" in Nineteenth Century Bengal'. In *Women and Culture*, edited by Kumkum Sangari and Sudesh Vaid, 103–12. Bombay: Research Centre for Women's Studies, 1994.

Saunders, Janet. 'The Magistrate and Madmen: Segregating the Criminally Insane in the Late Nineteenth Century Warwickshire'. In *Policing and Punishment in Nineteenth Century Britain*, edited by Victor Bailey, 217–41. London: Croom Helm, 1981.

Scull, Andrew. 'A Victorian Alienist: John Conolly, FRCP, DCL (1794–1866)'. In *The Anatomy of Madness: Essays in the History of Psychiatry, People and Ideas*, vol. 1, edited by W. F. Bynum, Roy Porter, and Michael Shephard, 103–51. London: Tavistock Publications, 1985.

Thomas, Mathew. 'Mental Hygiene as an International Movement'. In *International Health Organisations and Movements 1918–1939*, edited by Paul Weindling. Cambridge: Cambridge University Press, 1995.

Vaughan, Megan. 'Introduction'. In *Psychiatry and Empire*, edited by Sloan Mahone and Megan Vaughan. New York: Palgrave Macmillan, 2007.

Journal Articles

Andrews, Jonathan. 'Case Notes, Case Histories, and the Patient's Experience of Insanity at Gartnavel Royal Asylum, Glasgow, in the Nineteenth Century'. *Social History of Medicine*, vol. 11, no. 2 (1998).

Bagchi, Jasodhara. 'Representing Nationalism: Ideology of Motherhood in Colonial Bengal'. *Economic and Political Weekly*, vol. 25, nos 42/43 (1990): WS65–71.

Banerjee, Gauranga. 'First Psychiatric Clinic in a General Hospital in India'. *Mental Health Reviews* (2001). Available at http://www.psyplexus. com/excl/fpcg.html, accessed on 15 August 2012.

Basu, Amit Ranjan. 'Emergence of a Marginal Science in a Colonial City: Reading Psychiatry in Bengali Periodicals'. *Indian Economic and Social History Review*, vol. 41, no. 2 (2004).

Bhugra, Dinesh. 'Psychiatry in Ancient Indian Texts: A Review'. *History of Psychiatry*, vol. 3 (1992).

Broman, Thomas. 'Rethinking Professionalization: Theory, Practice, and Professional Ideology in Eighteenth-Century German Medicine'. *The Journal of Modern History*, vol. 67, no. 4 (1995).

Carroll, Michael P. 'The Folkloric Origin of Modern "Animal-Parented Children" Stories'. *Journal of Folklore Research*, vol. 21, no. 1 (April 1984).

Chatterton, C. '"Caught in the Middle"? Mental Nurse Training in England 1919–51'. *Journal of Psychiatric and Mental Health Nursing*, vol. 11, no. 1 (2004).

Cook, Harold J. 'Good Advice and Little Medicine: The Professional Authority of Early Modern English Physicians'. *Journal of British Studies*, vol. 33, no. 1 (1994): 1–31.

Dames, J. M. Longworth. 'Shah Daula's "Rats"'. *Man*, vol. 15 (1915).

Das, Debjani. 'Is Insanity a "*Female Malady*"? Lunatic Women in the Asylums of Bengal in the Nineteenth Century'. *Social Scientist*, vol. 39, nos 5–6 (May–June 2011).

Dhunjibhoy, Jal Edulji. 'A Brief Résumé of the Types of Insanity Commonly Met with in the Country India, with a Full Description of "Indian Hemp Insanity" Peculiar to the Country'. *Journal of Mental Sciences*, vol. 76 (1930).

Dols, Micheal W. 'Insanity and Its Treatment in Islamic Society'. *Medical History*, vol. 31 (1987).

Dreyer, Barbara A. 'Adolf Meyer and Mental Hygiene: An Ideal for Public Health'. *American Journal of Public Health*, vol. 66, no. 10 (1976).

Engels, Dagmar. 'The Age of Consent Act of 1891: Colonial Ideology in Bengal', *South Asia Research*, vol. 3, no. 2 (1983).

Ernst, Waltraud. 'Crossing the Boundaries of "Colonial Psychiatry": Reflections on the Development of Psychiatry in British India, c. 1870–1940'. *Culture, Medicine and Psychiatry*, vol. 35, no. 4 (December 2011).

———. 'Idioms of Madness and Colonial Boundaries: The Case of the European and "Native" Mentally Ill in Early Nineteenth-Century British India'. *Comparative Studies in Society and History*, vol. 39, no. 1 (1997).

———. 'The Indianization of Colonial Medicine: The Case of Psychiatry in Early-Twentieth Century British India'. *Journal of the History of Science, Technology and Medicine*, vol. 20, no. 4 (2012).

Gilani, Ahmed Ijaz, Umer Ijaz Gilani, Pashtoon Murtaza Kasi, and Murad Musa Khan. 'Psychiatric Health Laws in Pakistan: From Lunacy to Mental Health'. *Policy Forum*, vol. 2, no. 1 (2005).

Green, Nile. 'Breathing in India, c. 1890'. *Modern Asian Studies*, vol. 42, nos 2/3, (March–May, 2008).

———. 'Jack Sepoys and the Dervishes: Islam and the Indian Soldier in Princely India'. *Journal of Royal Asiatic Society*, vol. 18, no. 1 (2008).

Gupta, Charu. 'Procreation and Pleasure: Writings of a Woman Ayurvedic Practitioner in Colonial North India'. *Studies in History*, vol. 21, no. 1 (2005).

Huertas, Rafael, and C. M. Winston. 'Madness and Degeneration, I: From "Fallen Angel" to Mentally Ill'. *History of Psychiatry*, vol. 3, no. 4 (1992).

Jeffery, Roger. 'Recognizing India's Doctors: The Institutionalization of Medical Dependency'. *Modern Asian Studies*, vol. 13, no. 2 (1979).

Kala, Anirudh K., Alok Sarin, and Sanjeev Jain. 'The Psychiatrist's Partition'. *Himal South Asian*, vol. 20, no. 8 (August 2007).

Kapila, Shruti. 'Masculinity and Madness: Princely Personhood and Colonial Sciences of Mind in Western India, 1871–1940'. *Past and Present*, vol. 187, no. 1 (May 2005).

Kolsky, Elizabeth. 'Codification and the Rule of Colonial Difference: Criminal Procedure in British India'. *Law and History Review*, vol. 23, no. 3 (2005).

Kreisel, Deanna K. 'Wolf Children and Automata: Bestiality, Boredom at Home and Abroad'. *Representations*, vol. 96, no. 1 (2006).

Laws, Jennifer. 'Crackpots and Basket-Cases: A History of Therapeutic Work and Occupation'. *History of the Human Sciences*, vol. 24, no. 2 (2011).

Lloyd, Tom. 'Thuggee, Marginality and the State Effect in Colonial India, c. 1770–1840'. *Indian Economic and Social History Review*, vol. 45, no. 2 (2008).

Malcolm, Elizabeth 'Australian Asylum Architecture through German Eyes: Kew, Melbourne, 1867'. *Health and History*, vol. 11, no. 1 (2009).

Marks, Shula. 'What Is Colonial about Colonial Medicine? And What Happened to Imperialism and Health?'. *Social History of Medicine*, vol. 10, no. 2 (1997).

McCrae, Niall. "'A Violent Thunderstorm": Cardiazol Treatment in British Mental Hospitals'. *History of Psychiatry*, vol. 17, no. 1 (2006).

Miles, M. 'Pakistan's Microcephalic Chuas of Shah Daulah: Cursed, Clamped or Cherished?'. *History of Psychiatry*, vol. 7 (1996).

Mills, James H. 'The History of Modern Psychiatry in India, 1858–1947'. *History of Psychiatry*, vol. 12, no. 4 (2001).

———. 'Reforming the Indian: Treatment Regimes in the Lunatic Asylums of British India, 1857–1880'. *Indian Economic Social History Review*, vol. 36, no. 4 (1999).

Moran, Richard. 'The Modern Foundation for the Insanity Defence: The Cases of James Hadfield (1800) and Daniel McNaughtan (1843)'. *American Academy of Political and Social Science*, vol. 447, no. 1 (1985).

Mukharji, Projit B. 'Vernacularizing the Body: Informational Egalitarianism, Hindu Divine Design and Race in Physiology School Books, Bengal 1859–1877'. *Bulletin of the History of Medicine*, vol. 91, no. 3 (2107).

Nizame, S. Haque, and Nishant Goyal. 'History of Psychiatry in India'. *Indian Journal of Psychiatry*, vol. 52, no. 1 (2010).

Patch, Charles Lodge. 'Microcephaly: A Report on "The Shah Daulah's Mice"'. *Indian Medical Gazette*, vol. 63 (1928).

Prestwich, Patricia E. 'Family Strategies and Medical Power: "Voluntary" Committals in a Parisian Asylum, 1876–1914'. *Journal of Social History*, vol. 27, no. 4 (1994).

Radhakranshna, Meena. 'Of Apes and Ancestors: Evolutionary Science and Colonial Ethnography'. *The Indian Historical Review*, vol. 33, no. 1 (January 2006).

Rajpal, Shilpi. 'Colonial Psychiatry in Mid-Nineteenth Century: The James Clark Enquiry'. *South Asia Research*, vol. 35, no. 1 (February 2015).

———. 'Experiencing the Indian Archives'. *Economic and Political Weekly*, vol. 47, no. 16 (April 2012).

———. 'Quotidian Madness: Time, Management and Asylums in Colonial North India, c. 1850–1947'. *Studies in History*, vol. 31, no. 1 (August 2015).

Ranganathan, Shubha. 'Healing Temples, the Anti-Superstition Discourse and Global Mental Health: Some Questions from Mahanubhav Temples in India'. *South Asia: Journal of South Asian Studies*, vol. 37, no. 4 (2014).

Rollin, Henry R. 'Psychiatry in Britain One Hundred Years Ago'. *The British Journal of Psychiatry*, vol. 183, no. 10 (2003).

Saha, Jonathan. 'Madness and the Making of a Colonial Order in Burma'. *Modern Asian Studies*, vol. 47, no. 2 (2013).

Sarkar, Sumit. "'Kaliyuga", "Chakri" and "Bhakti": Ramakrishna and His Times'. *Economic and Political Weekly*, vol. 27, no. 29 (18 July 1992).

Sarkar, Tanika. 'A Prehistory of Rights: The Age of Consent Debate in Colonial Bengal', *Feminist Studies*, vol. 26, no. 3 (2000).

———. 'Rhetoric against Age of Consent: Resisting Colonial Reason and Death of a Child-Wife'. *Economic and Political Weekly*, vol. 28, no. 36 (1993).

Scott, James C. 'Everyday Forms of Resistance'. *Copenhagen Journal of Asian Studies*, vol. 67, no. 4 (1989).

Scull, Andrew. 'Somatic Treatments and the Historiography of Psychiatry'. *History of Psychiatry*, vol. 5, no. 1 (1994).

Sen, Indrani. 'The Memsahib's "Madness": The European Woman's Mental Health in Late Nineteenth Century India'. *Social Scientist*, vol. 33, nos 5–6 (May–June 2005).

Sen, Satadru. 'The Savage Family: Colonialism and Female Infanticide in Nineteenth Century India'. *Journal of Women's History*, vol. 14, no. 3 (2002).

Shah, Shalini. 'Representation of Female Sexuality in the Ayurvedic Discourse of the Early Medieval Period'. *Studies in History*, vol. 22, no. 1 (2006).

Sivramakrishnan, Kavita. 'Constructing Boundaries, Contesting Identities: The Politics of Ayurved in Punjab (1930–1940)'. *Studies in History*, vol. 22, no. 2 (2006).

Sommer, Andreas. 'Psychical Research in the History and Philosophy of Science: An Introduction and Review'. *Studies in History and Philosophy of Biological and Biomedical Sciences*, vol. 48 (2014).

Stoler, Ann Laura. 'Making Empire Respectable: The Politics of Race and Sexual Morality in 20th-Century Colonial Cultures'. *American Ethnologist*, vol. 16, no. 4 (1989).

Swartz, Sally. 'Colonizing the Insane: Causes of Insanity in the Cape'. *History of the Human Sciences*, vol. 8, no. 4 (1995).

Thomson, E. P. 'Time, Work-Discipline and Industrial Capitalism'. *Past and Present*, vol. 38, no. 1 (1967).

Unsworth, Clive. 'Law and Lunacy in Psychiatry's "Golden Age"'. *Oxford Journal of Legal Studies*, vol. 13, no. 4 (1993).

Vaughan, Megan. 'Idioms of Madness: Zomba Lunatic Asylum, Nyasaland, in the Colonial Period'. *Journal of Southern African Studies*, vol. 9, no. 2 (April 1983): 218–38.

Vishwanath, L. S. 'Efforts of Colonial State to Suppress Female Infanticide: Use of Sacred Texts, Generation of Knowledge'. *Economic and Political Weekly*, vol. 33, no. 19 (May 1998).

Wagner, Kim. 'The Deconstructed Stranglers: A Reassessment of Thuggee'. *Modern Asian Studies*, vol. 38, no. 4 (2004).

Walter, Richard D. 'What Became of the Degenerate? A Brief History of a Concept'. *Journal of the History of Medicine and the Allied Sciences*, vol. 11, no. 4 (1956).

Wright, David, and A. Shepherd. 'Madness, Suicide and the Victorian Asylum: Attempted Self-Murder in the Age of Non Restraint'. *Medical History*, vol. 46, no. 2 (2002).

York, Sarah. 'Alienists, Attendants and the Containment of Suicide in Public Lunatic Asylums, 1845–1890'. *Social History of Medicine*, vol. 25, no. 2 (2012).

Zysk, Kenneth G. 'Potency Therapy in Classical Indian Medicine'. *Asian Medicine*, vol. 1, no. 1 (2005).

Newspaper Articles

Venkatesan, J. 'SC Issues Notice to States, Centre on Condition of Mental Hospitals'. *The Hindu*, 9 July 2013.

Unpublished Dissertation

Bhattacharyya, Anouska. 'Indian Insanes: Lunacy in the "Native" Asylums of Colonial India, 1858–1912'. Doctoral thesis submitted to Harvard University, Cambridge, 2013.

Kapila, Shruti. 'The Making of Colonial Psychiatry, Bombay Presidency, 1849–1940'. Doctoral thesis submitted to School of Oriental and African Studies, University of London, 2002.

Pinto, Sarah Ann. 'Shackled Bodies, Unchained Minds: Lunatic Asylums in Bombay Presidency, 1793–1921'. Doctoral thesis submitted to Victoria University of Wellington, 2017.

Rajpal, Shilpi. '"Madness" and Delinquency in Colonial North India, c.1850–1947'. Doctoral thesis submitted to University of Delhi, 2014.

Raveendranathan, Vidhya. 'Constructing the Scavenger: Caste and Labour in Colonial South India, 1860–1940'. MPhil. dissertation submitted to University of Delhi, 2011.

Saha, Ranjana. 'Modern Maternities: Discourses on Breastfeeding and Child Development in Colonial Bengal'. Unpublished PhD thesis, University of Delhi, 2017.

Weiss, Mitchell G. 'Critical Study of Unmada in Early Sanskrit Literature: An Analysis of Ayurvedic Psychiatry with Reference to Present-day Diagnostic Concepts'. Doctoral thesis submitted to University of Pennsylvania, 1977.

Index

About the Author

Shilpi Rajpal teaches at the School of Liberal Arts, Surat, India. She was previously an assistant professor in the Department of History and Culture, Jamia Milia Islamia, New Delhi. She was awarded the Charles Wallace India Trust Research Grant in 2015. She was a postdoctoral fellow in the Department of Humanities and Social Sciences, Indian Institute of Science Education and Research, Mohali. Her work has been published in journals such as *The Indian Economic and Social History Review*, *Studies in History*, and *South Asia Research*.